CURING YOGA

100+ HEALING YOGA SEQUENCES TO
ALLEVIATE OVER 50 AILMENTS

AVENTURAS DE VIAJE

Illustrated by
OKIANG LUHUNG

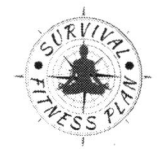

CONTENTS

POSES

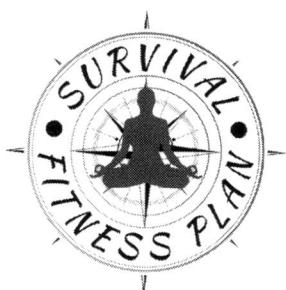

WARNINGS AND DISCLAIMERS

The information in this publication is made public for reference only.

Neither the author, publisher, nor anyone else involved in the production of this publication is responsible for how the reader uses the information or the result of his/her actions.

Consult a physician before undertaking any new form of physical activity.

HOW TO USE THIS BOOK

Besides the chapters on breathing and Yoga Nidra, this book is split into 2 main parts.

Sequences

In this section you will find all the yoga sequences for increasing your energy.

Each sequence has images and a list of poses which make up the sequence.

The list of poses correlate to the images with the first pose starting at the top left and the last finishing at the bottom right.

For those of you familiar with basic yoga poses you can see and do all the poses in the sequence at a glance.

For everyone else there is part 2 of the book.

Poses

This section contains instructions on how to do all the poses mentioned in the sequences.

They are in alphabetical order for easy reference.

BREATHING

There are a few different types of breathing methods in yoga, but for all the routines in this book we only use two basic ones.

Three Part Breath

This is the breath you will use most often when practicing yoga. Use it while doing the sequences in this book.

When first learning it you will probably just want to do it from a sitting or lying position.

Breathe in long and deep through your nose. First feel it enter your lower belly, then your lower chest/rib cage, and finally into your lower throat/top of sternum. Feel the clear, positive energies of love and happiness come up from your toes to you head.

When you are ready exhale fully through your nose, feeling it leave in the opposite order it came in, i.e., first in your sternum, then your chest, and finally your belly. Release all tension and negative energies out of your body from your head to your toes.

Continue to breathe in and out like this, smooth and continuous.

When you first start to practice this type of breathing it may help to put your hands on each of the three areas as you do it, i.e. belly, chest, and sternum. You can also try just breathing into each area on its own.

Alternate Nostril Breathing

Alternate nostril breathing is a quick and easy way to calm your nervous system and raise your happiness. It also helps clear congestion.

Sit tall and comfortable.

Curl down your middle and index fingers of your right hand into your palm.

Press your right ring finger on your left nostril to close it and breathe in to the count of four.

Now use your thumb to close off your right nostril so both your nostrils are closed. Count to four.

Release your ring finger and breathe out through your left nostril to the count of four.

Repeat this same sequence but now breathe in through your right nostril.

Continue this alternation for 3 to 5 minutes.

YOGA NIDRA

Yoga Nidra is a form of guided meditation which has many health benefits. You can guide yourself but the easiest way to do it is to listen to a Yoga Nidra practice and do what the instructor says.

For best results find a place where your body can be comfortable and you can practice undisturbed. Not too hot or cold. Put on some soothing background music if you want.

It is best not to do Yoga Nidra in bed because you will be more likely to fall asleep. A yoga mat on the floor is ideal.

Yoga Nidra is a conscious practice.

Lie in Corpse Pose

Corpse pose, a.k.a. Shavasana, is a yoga pose used at the end of almost every yoga practice. Going straight from your yoga practice to Yoga Nidra is ideal and is (in my opinion) most likely the intention of the ones who created it.

Yoga Nidra can also be done from a seated position if lying down is inappropriate.

Close your eyes.

Corpse pose is explained in detail in the Poses section of this book.

Notice your Breath

Notice your breathing. Feel your lungs filling with air, your stomach expanding, and then deflating.

Imagine a light around your body expanding and contracting as you breathe in and out.

Feel the energy coursing through your body.

Use Your Senses

Notice each of your senses individually.

What sounds do you hear? Near, far, inside, outside.

What smells can you smell? Take small sniffs, like a dog does.

Taste the air.

Feel your body supported on the floor. Which parts of your body are touching?

What can you see with your eyes closed? Does the light make shapes in your eyelids?

Repeat Your Mantra

Your mantra is a short sentence stating your intentions. It's kind of like an affirmation. It may be an overall statement of health, relaxation, etc., or may be a visualization of something you want to achieve.

Whatever it is, repeat it mentally three times. Try to feel how it feels as if the visualization was realized.

One I use often is "My entire being is completely relaxed and at one with the universe."

Scan Your Body

This is where you consciously relax each part of your body.

Mentally go through your body. Bring your attention to and relax each part. You can be very detailed about this or just do large areas. It depends on how long you want to spend.

I start from the top of my head and work my way down. Sometimes I even do internal organs.

After you have relaxed smaller body parts relax them as a whole, e.g., shoulder, upper arm, bicep, elbow, forearm, hand, fingers, relax the whole arm.

At the end relax the whole body as one.

Awaken the Body

The last step is to slowly deepen your breath and start to move your fingers and toes, then your hands and feet.

In your own time stretch out your body out however feels right. Open your eyes when you are ready.

When you are done stretching gently hug your knees (wind relieving pose). Fall to your right side and then gently sit up.

Take a moment to reflect on the practice and then go about your day.

SEQUENCES

How long each of these sequences take is up to you. Stay in each pose for as long as you desire.

While doing the sequences use deep breathing such as three part breath. It is a very important part of yoga.

Unless otherwise stated (such as in the circulation sequence), when doing a pose on one side also do it on the opposite side in immediate succession.

If you do not know how to do a pose you can learn how to do it in the Poses section of this book.

Note: If you ever find yourself in a painful position, back out of it slowly to avoid injury.

ACHES & PAINS

This is a very general sequence to help with mild body aches and pains.

Be sure to breathe, move slowly, and pay attention to what your body is telling you.

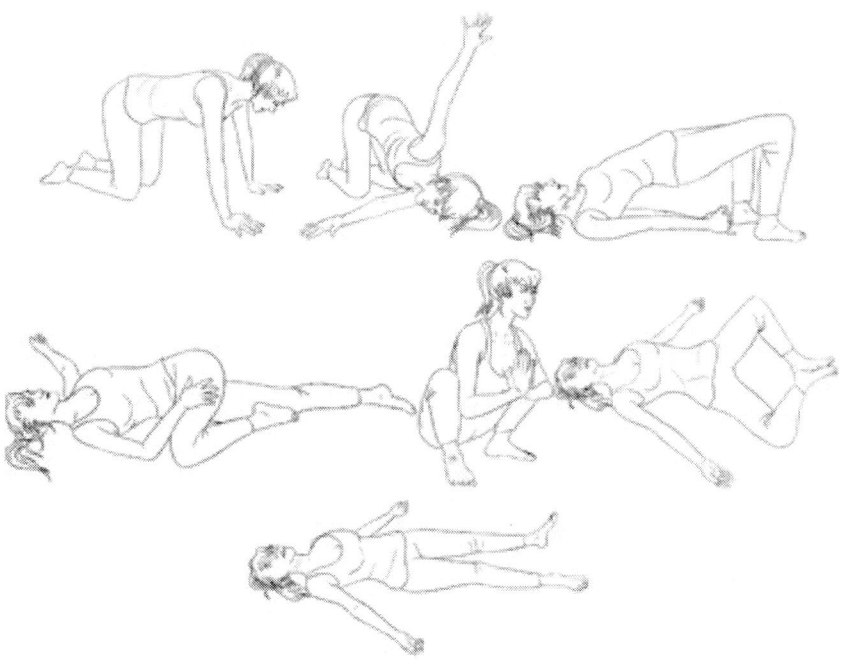

Table - Threading the Needle – Bridge Knee Down Twist - Prayer Squat - Supine Bound Angle Corpse

ACNE

Try this routine daily and eat a healthy diet for best results.

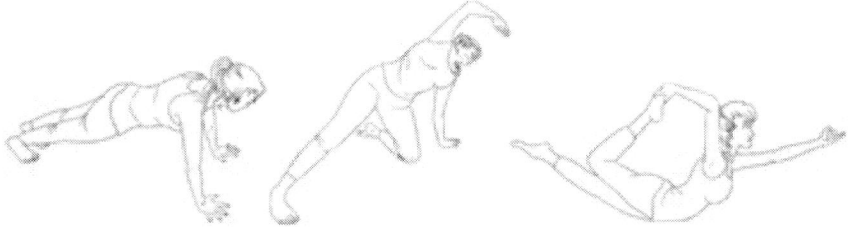

Plank - Half Circle - Half Bow

ADD / ADHD

These quick routines are also good for anybody with a cluttered mind, such as after an extra hard day at work.

ADD / ADHD SEQUENCE ONE

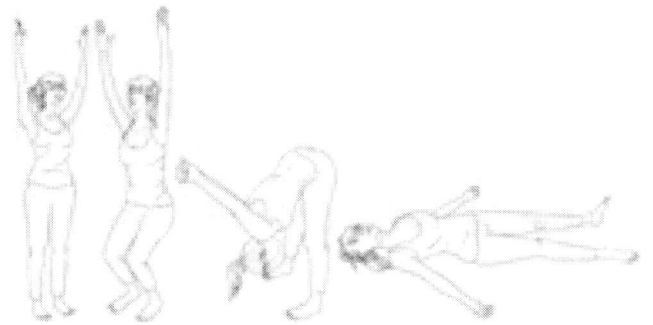

ADD/ADHD Sequence One: Mountain – Chair - Standing Yoga Seal – Corpse

ADD/ADHD SEQUENCE TWO
Seated Spinal Twist – Tree

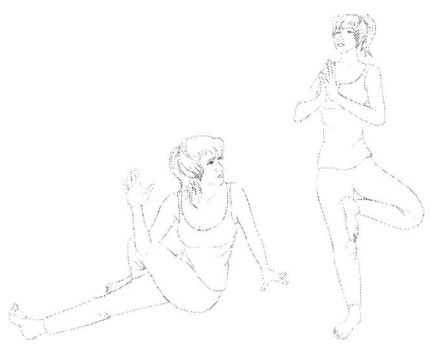

Seated Spinal Twist – Tree

ALLERGIES

Do this routine twice daily when you experience symptoms of allergy.

This sequence is also good to do at least three times a week for building up your general immunity.

Also see the sequences for cold and flu, and immunity.

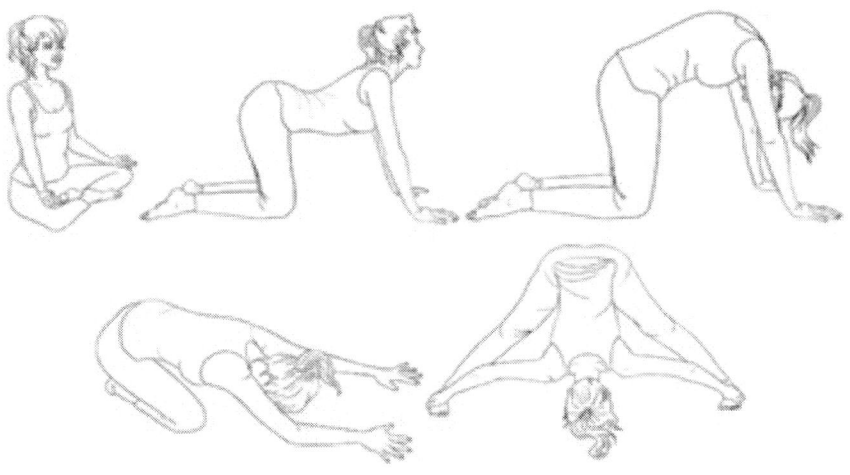

Accomplished (with alternate nostril breathing) - Dog Tilt - Cat Tilt - Child - Wide Legged Forward Bend

ARTHRITIS

The following sequence is very general. You may wish to add poses depending on your problem area.

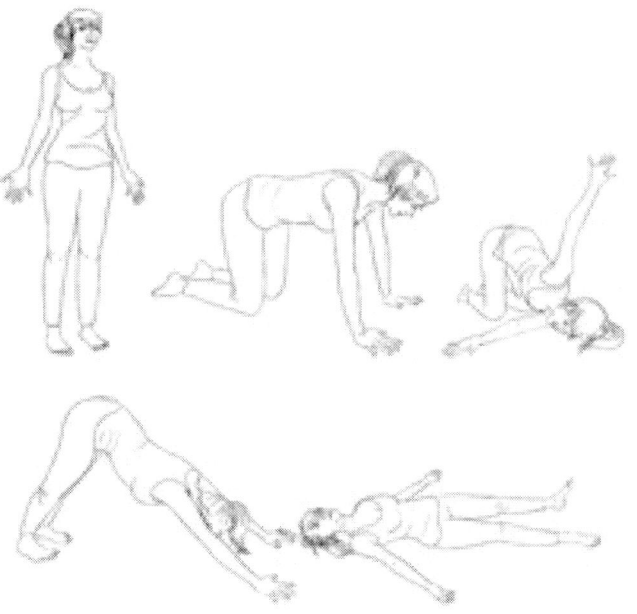

Mountain – Table - Threading the Needle Downward Dog –
Corpse

ASTHMA

While doing this sequence pay special attention to opening your chest.

Also see the respiratory ailments sequence.

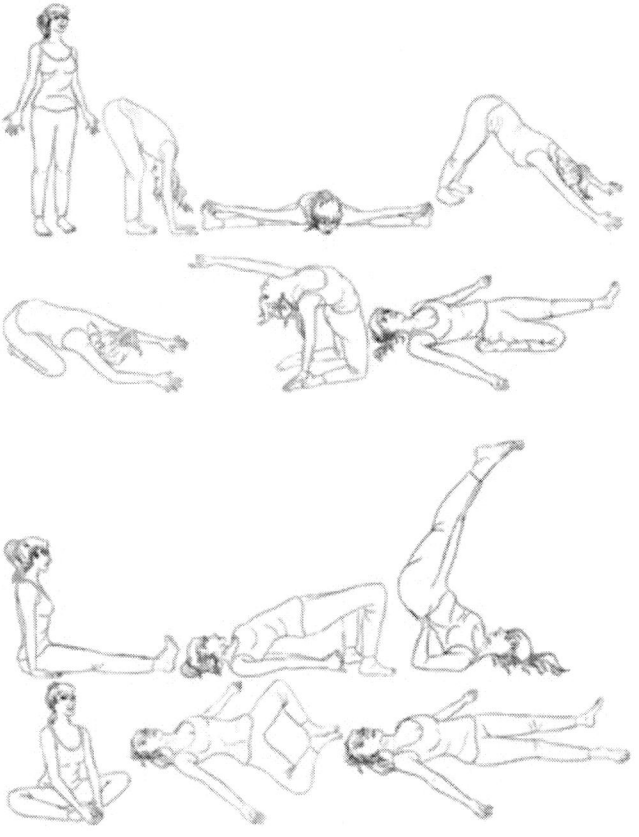

Mountain – Standing Forward Fold - Seated Angle - Downward Dog - Child - Half Camel - Half Supine Hero - Staff – Bridge - Half Shoulder-stand - Bound Angle - Supine Bound Angle – Corpse

BACKACHE

Be very careful when doing sequences for backache. Move slowly, never strain or hold your breath, and keep your neck and facial muscles relaxed.

BACKACHE SEQUENCE ONE

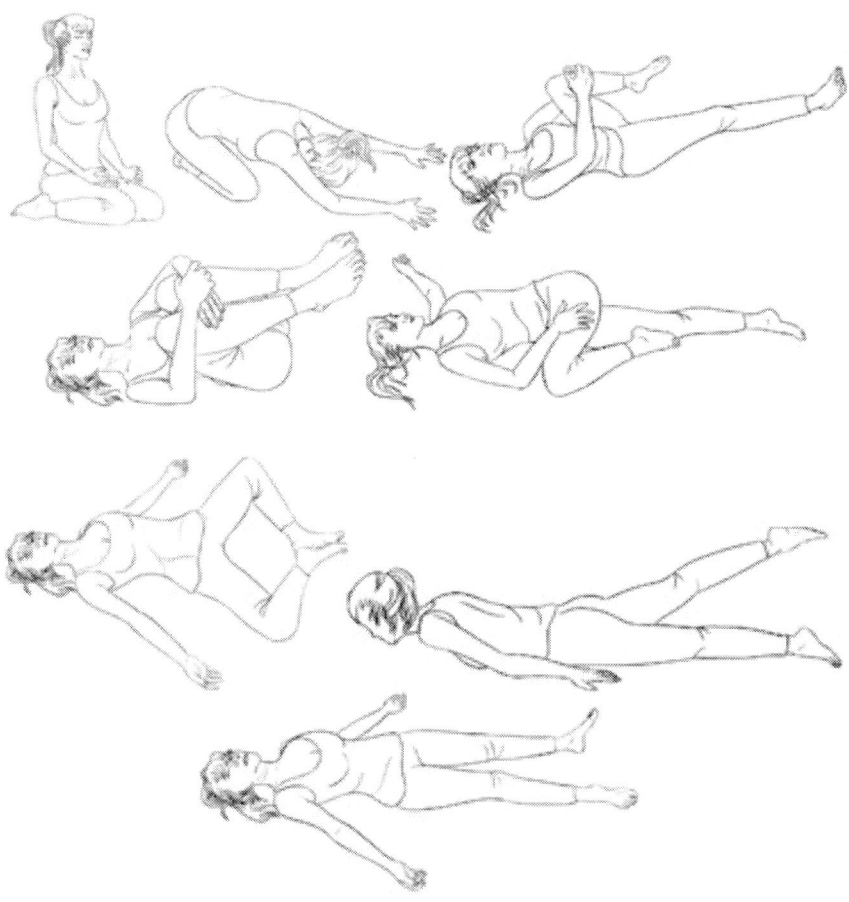

*Hero – Child - Half Wind Relieving - Wind Relieving - Knee Down Twist - Supine
Bound Angle - Half Locust - Corpse*

BACKACHE SEQUENCE TWO

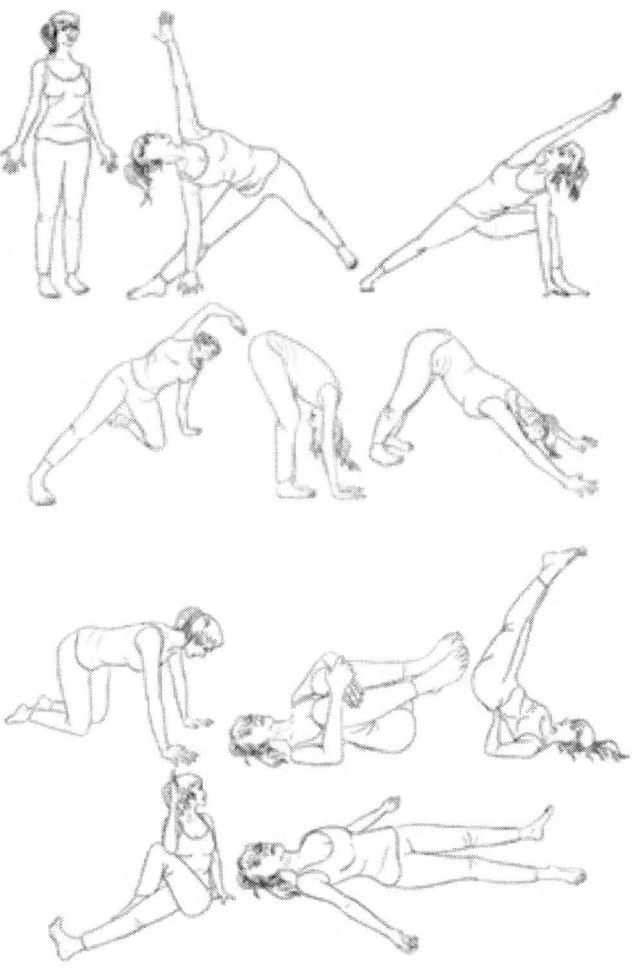

Mountain – Triangle - Extended Side Angle - Half Circle -
Standing Forward Fold - Downward Dog - Table - Wind
Relieving - Half Shoulder Stand - Seated Spinal Twist – Corpse

BACKACHE SEQUENCE THREE

This sequence is specifically helpful for the upper back and neck.

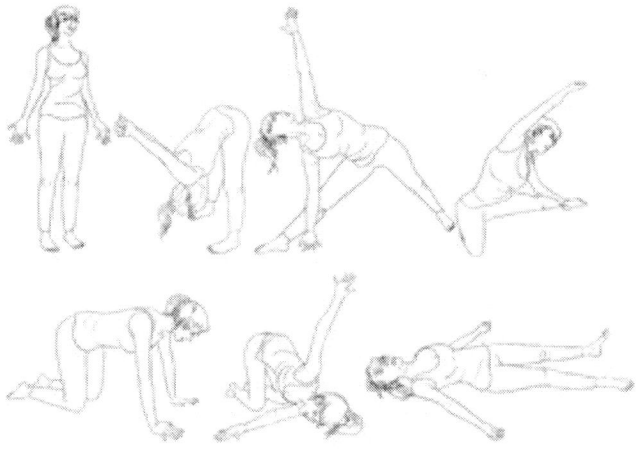

Mountain - Standing Yoga Seal – Triangle – Gate - Table -
Threading the Needle – Corpse

BALANCE

This sequence improves balance in your mind and body.

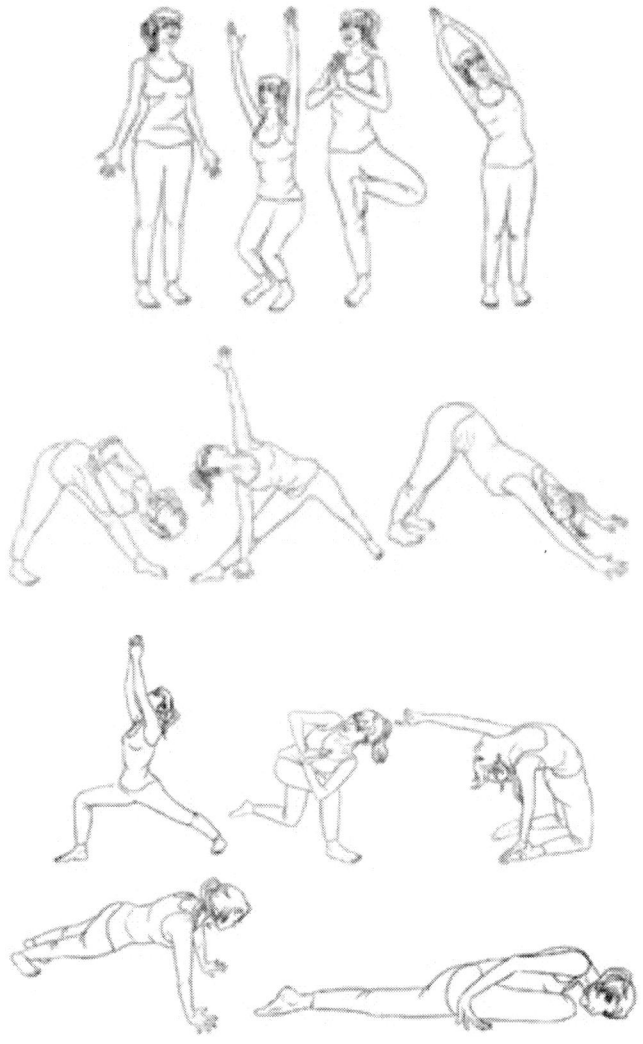

Mountain – Chair – Tree – Crescent Moon - Pyramid – Triangle
- Downward Dog - Warrior One - Half Prayer Twist - Half
Camel - Plank – Extended Pigeon

BROKEN HEART

When you feel broken hearted, do this sequence daily until you feel better.

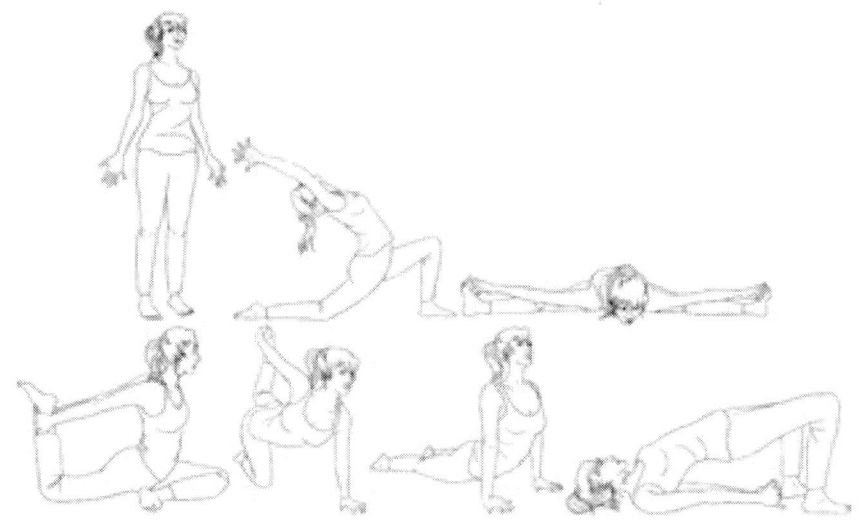

Mountain - Low Warrior - Seated Angle - Pigeon - One Handed Tiger - Upward Dog – Bridge

CHANGE

This sequence will help you adjust to times of change in all areas of life.

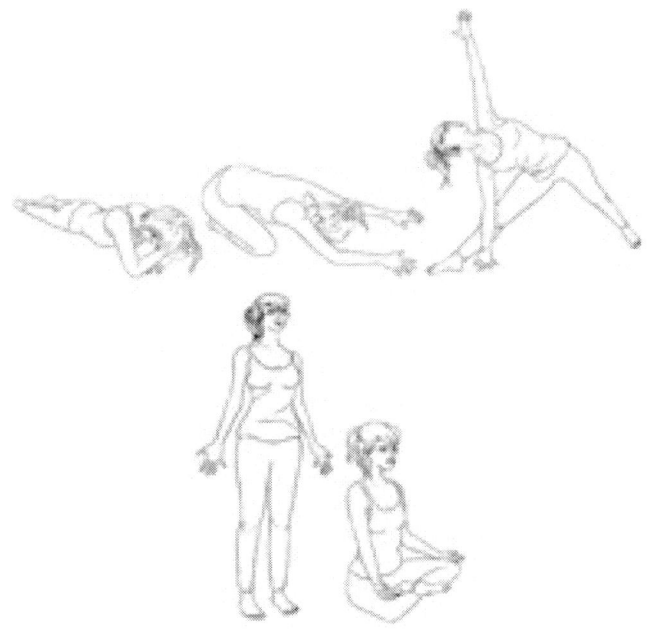

Crocodile – Child – Triangle - Mountain - Accomplished (with meditation)

CIRCULATION

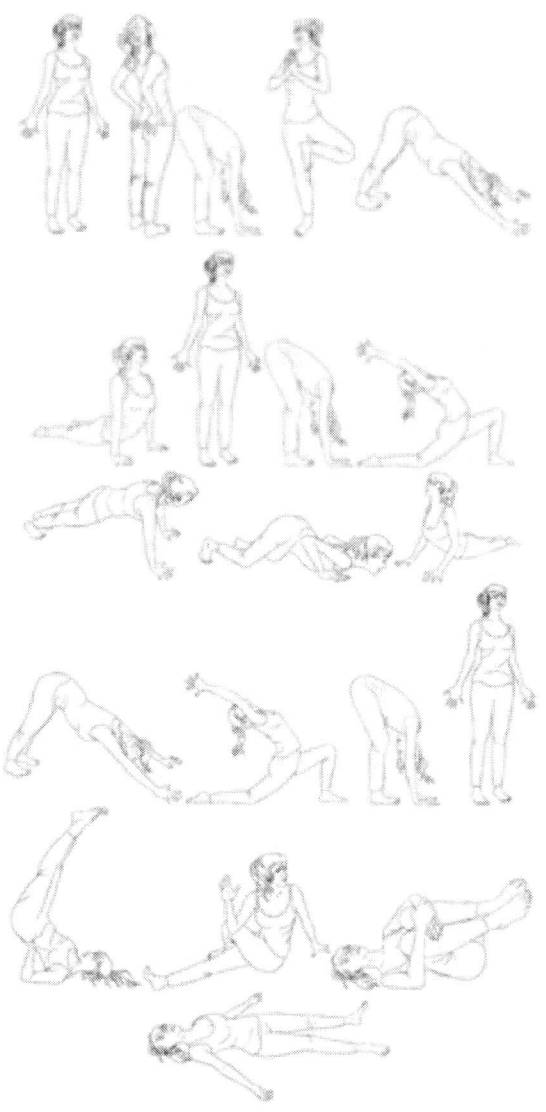

Mountain - Standing Backbend – Standing Forward Fold – Tree - Downward Dog - Upward Dog – Mountain – Standing Forward Fold - Low Warrior (right side) - Plank – Caterpillar – Cobra - Downward Dog - Low Warrior (left side) – Standing Forward Fold – Mountain - Half Shoulder-stand – Seated Spinal Twist – Wind Relieving - Corpse

COLD AND FLU

Both of these sequences are useful for cure and prevention of colds since they also strengthen your immune system in general.

While doing these sequences pay special attention to opening your chest.

Also see the sequences for allergy and immunity.

COLD AND FLU SEQUENCE ONE

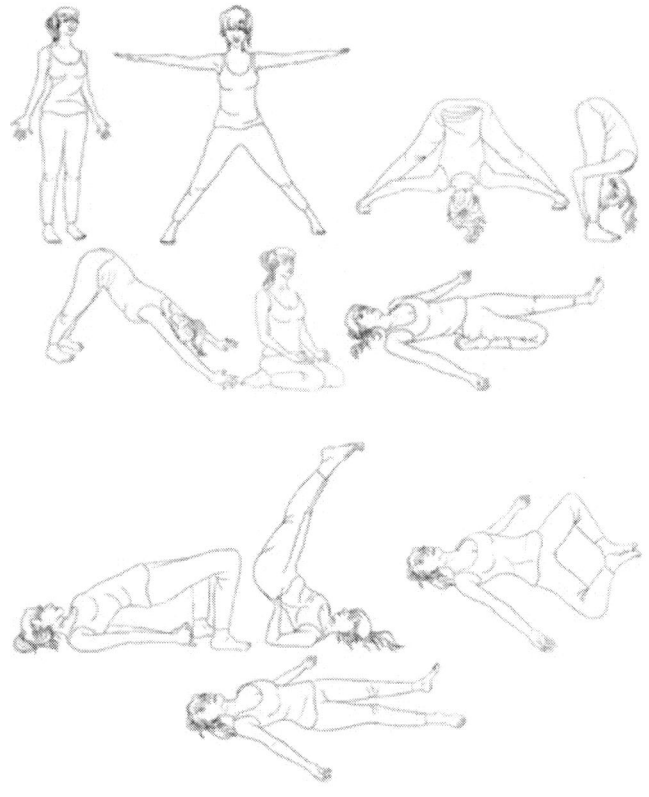

Mountain - Five pointed star – Wide Legged Forward Bend -
Standing Forward Fold - Downward Dog – Hero - Half Supine
Hero - Bridge - Half Shoulder-stand - Supine Bound Angle -
Corpse

COLD AND FLU SEQUENCE TWO

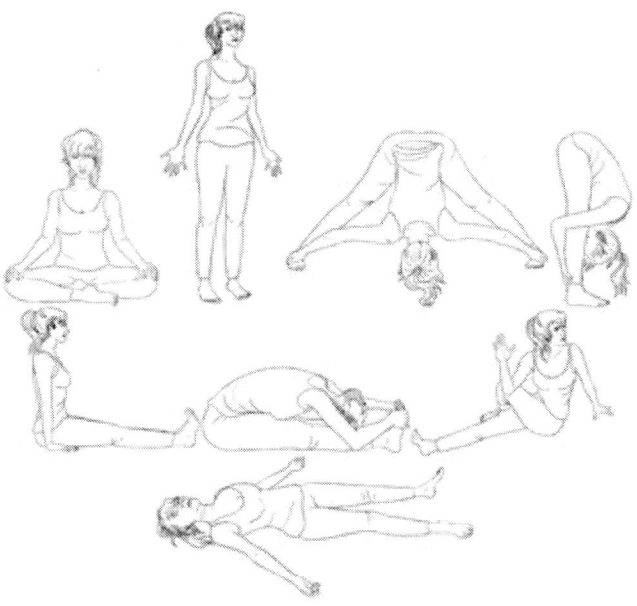

Accomplished (with alternate nostril breathing) – Mountain -
Wide Legged Forward Bend - Standing Forward Fold - Staff -
Seated Head to Knee - Seated Spinal Twist Corps

COMPLEXION

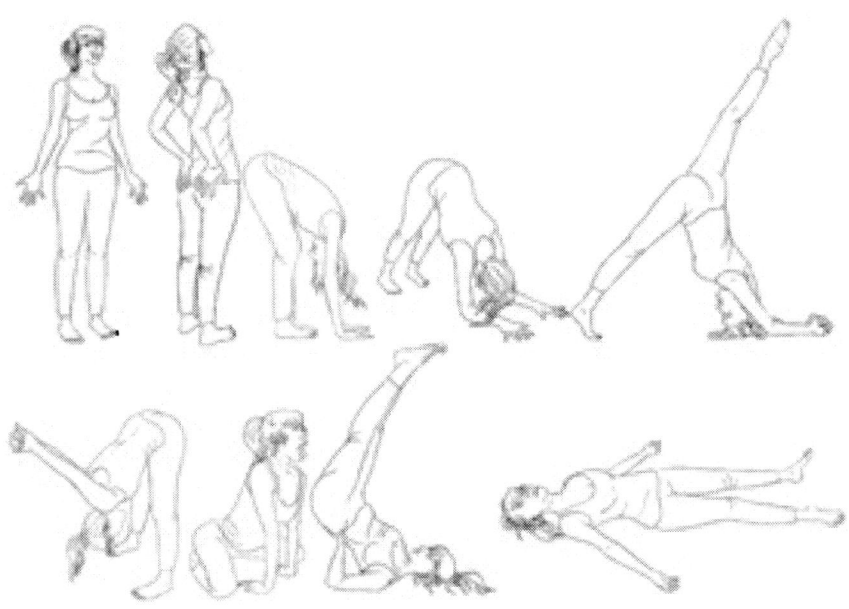

Mountain - Standing Backbend - Standing Forward Fold – Dolphin - One Legged Dolphin - Standing Yoga Seal – Lion - Half Shoulder-stand – Corpse

CRAVINGS

Whatever's your craving or addiction (alcohol, cigarettes, drugs, sugar, etc.) this sequence can help.

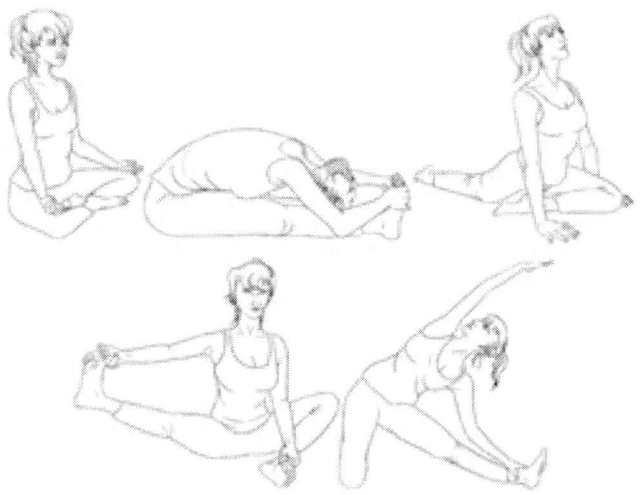

Accomplished - Seated Forward Bend – Pigeon - Half Upright
Seated Angle – Gate

DEPRESSION

Any of these sequences can be used for long-term depression or even just a quick "pick-me-up" when you are feeling a little down.

DEPRESSION SEQUENCE ONE

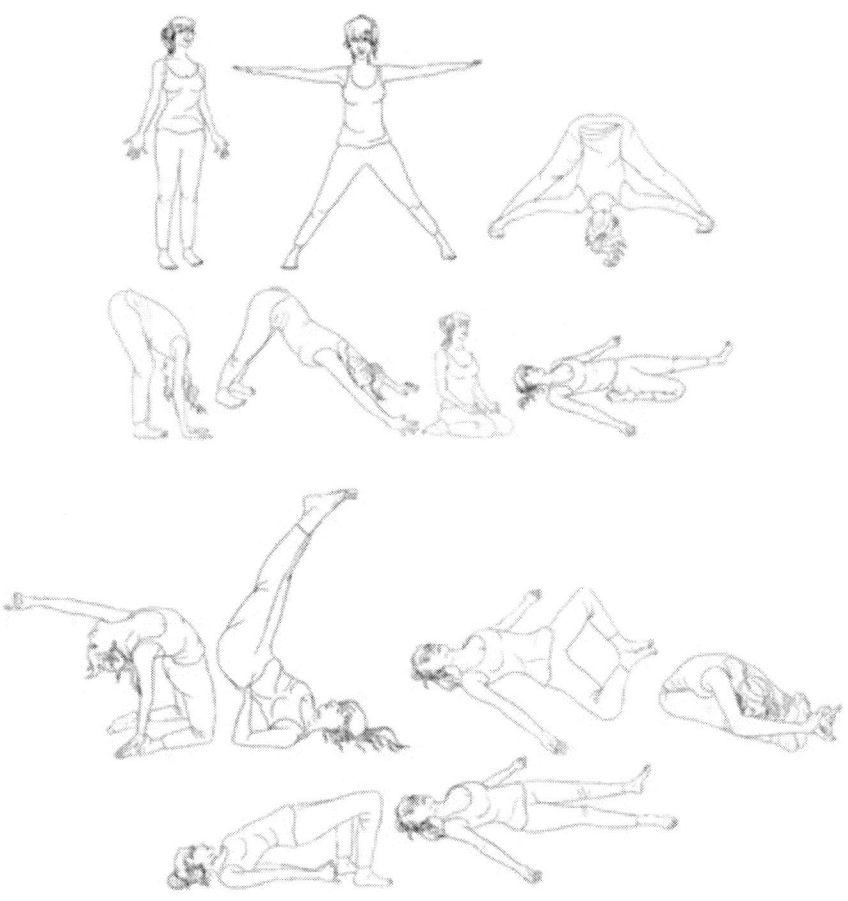

Mountain - Five Pointed Star – Wide Legged Forward Bend - Standing Forward Fold - Downward Dog – Hero - Half Supine Hero - Half Camel - Half Shoulderstand - Supine Bound Angle - Seated Forward Bend - Bridge – Corpse

DEPRESSION SEQUENCE TWO

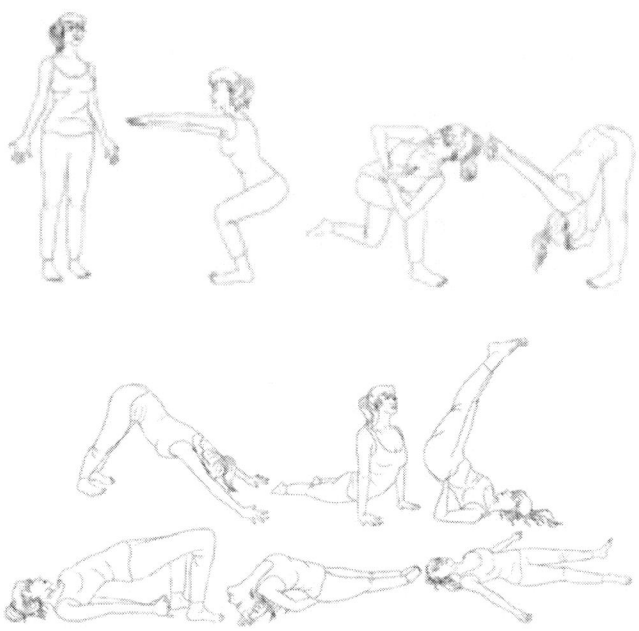

Mountain – Chair - Low Warrior - Half Prayer Twist - Standing Yoga Seal - Downward Dog - Upward Dog - Half Shoulder-stand - Fish – Bridge – Corpse

DEPRESSION SEQUENCE THREE

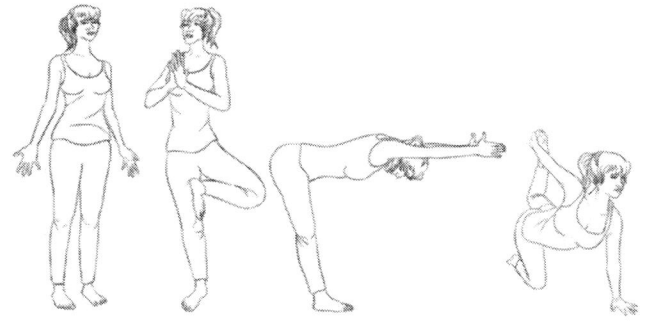

Mountain - Tree - Half Forward Fold – One Handed Tiger

DEPRESSION SEQUENCE FOUR

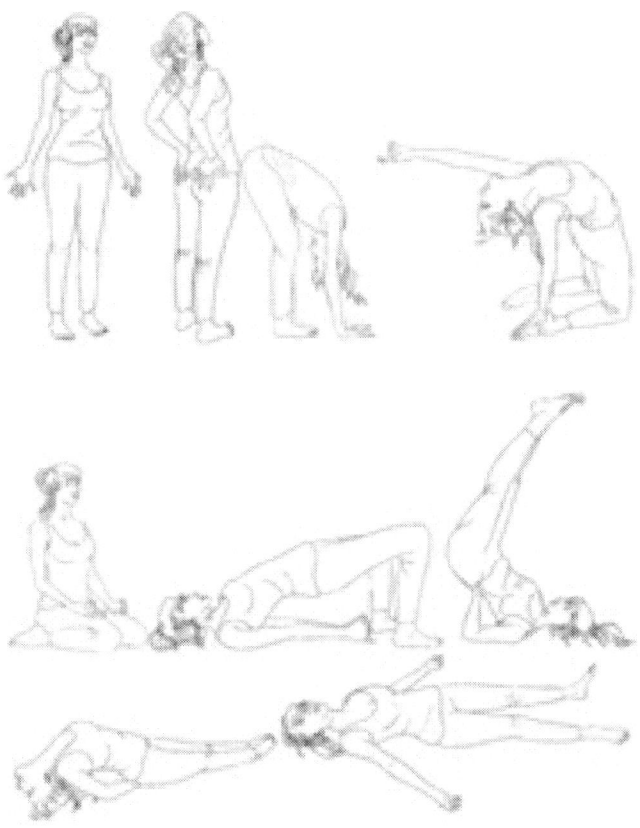

*Mountain - Standing Back Bend – Standing Forward Fold - Half
Camel - Hero – Bridge - Half Shoulder-stand - Fish – Corpse*

FIBROMYALGIA

When doing this sequence paying attention to your breath is especially important. Also concentrate on relaxing your muscles.

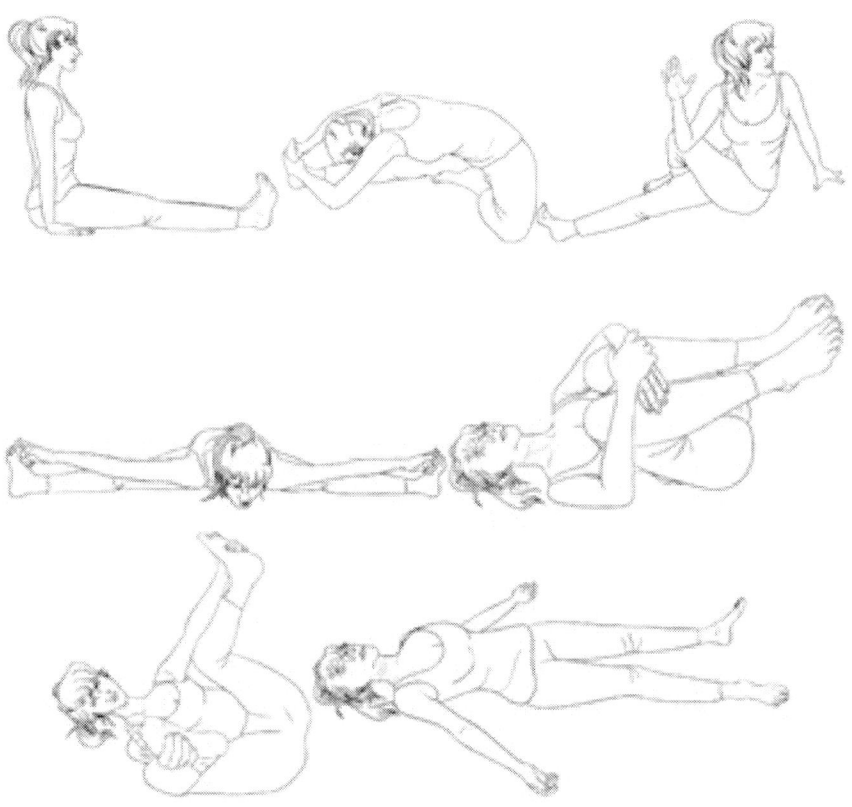

Staff - Seated Head to Knee - Seated Spinal Twist - Seated Angle - Wind Relieving
- Joyful Baby – Corpse

FOOT CRAMPS

To soothe a sudden onset of foot cramps, squat down and sit on your heels with your toes tucked.

If you have a bit more time use the following sequence which also helps for prevention when done a few times a week.

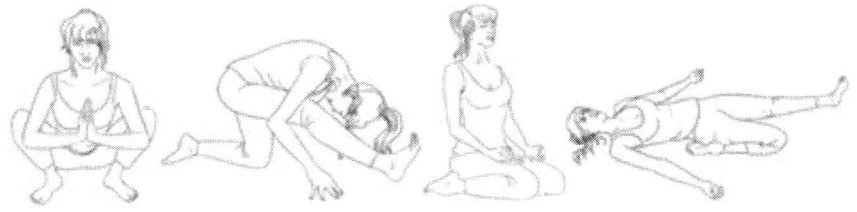

Prayer Squat (on balls of feet) - Half Pyramid – Hero - Half Supine Hero

HANGOVER

Handstands are not included in this book as they are considered more than a basic pose, but they are great for headaches and hangovers, so if you can, do them.

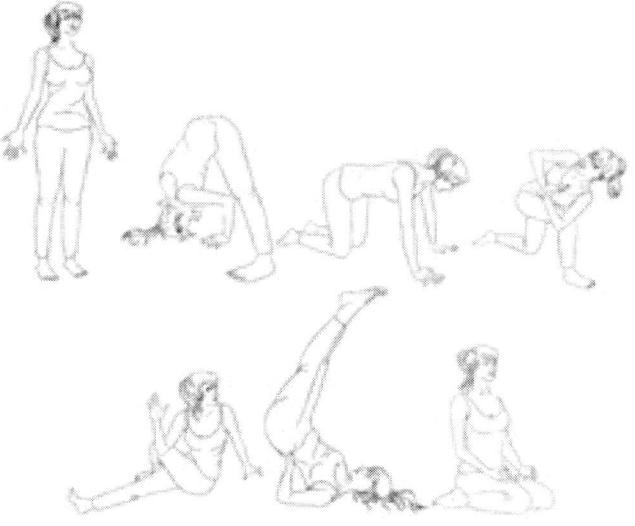

Mountain – Wide Legged Forward Bend – Table - Half Prayer Twist - Seated Spinal Twist - Half Shoulder-stand – Hero

HEADACHE AND MIGRAINE

The following sequences are good for the "everyday" headache as well as chronic migraines.

They can also be done regularly to help keep migraines away for good.

When doing these sequences focus on keeping your brain quiet and lengthening the neck.

HEADACHE/MIGRAINE SEQUENCE ONE

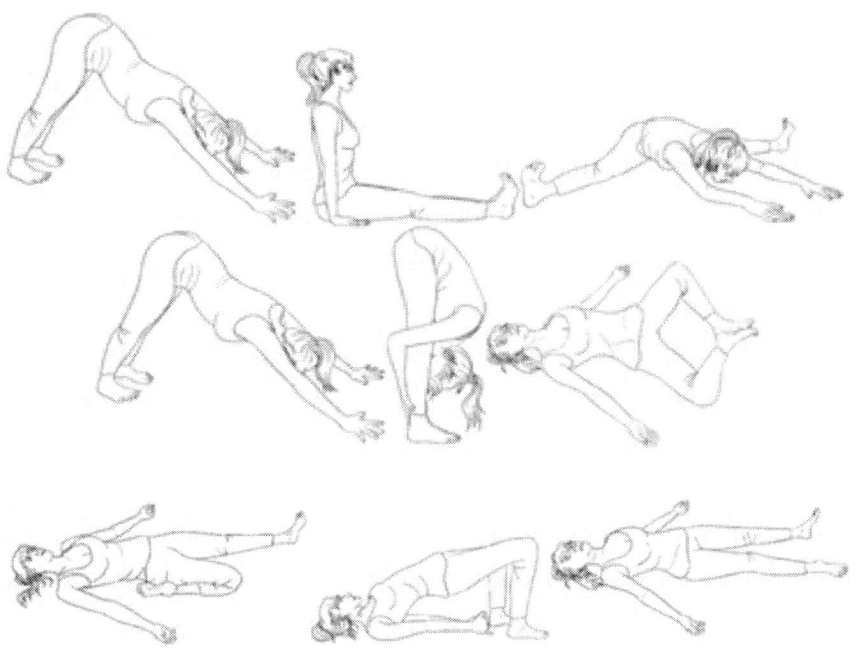

Downward Dog – Staff - Seated Forward Bend - Seated Angle - Downward Dog - Standing Forward Fold - Supine Bound Angle - Half Supine Hero – Bridge – Corpse

HEADACHE/MIGRAINE SEQUENCE TWO

To do the temple massage use your index fingers to press on your third eye then trace a two opposing lines with your fingers to your temples. Repeat this several times.

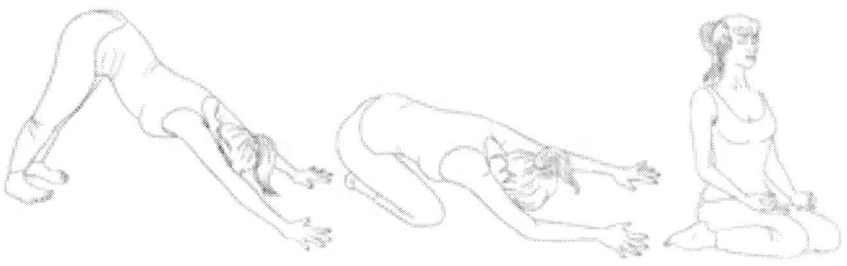

Downward Dog – Child - Hero (with temple massage)

HEART AND LUNGS

This sequence is not for any specific ailment but will help to strengthen your heart and lungs in general.

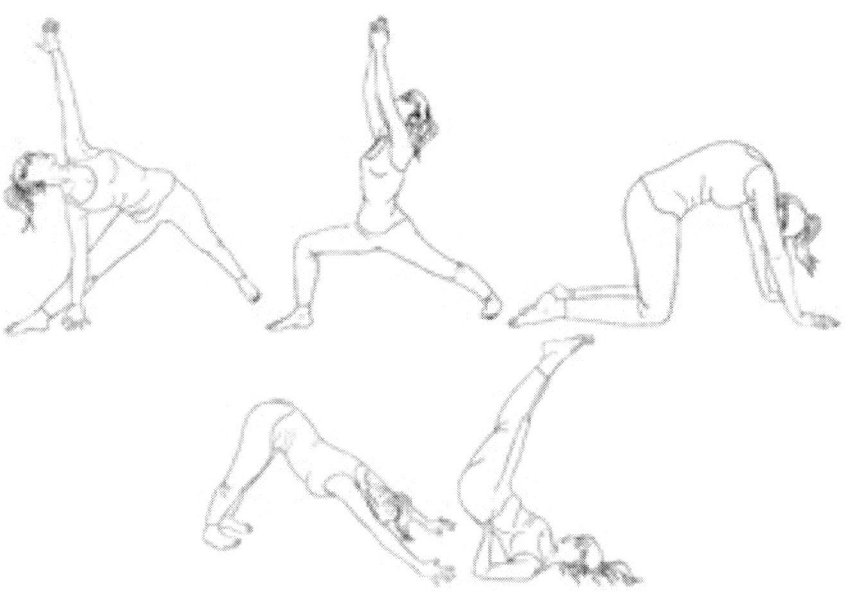

Triangle - Warrior One – Cat Tilt – Cobra - Downward Dog - Half Shoulder-stand

HIGH BLOOD PRESSURE

If you have high blood pressure be sure to check with your physician before starting any new exercise regime, including yoga.

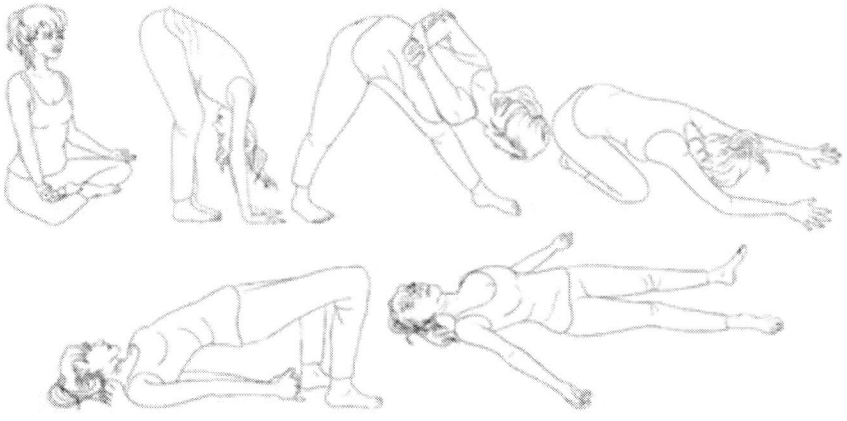

Accomplished (with alternate nostril breathing) - Standing Forward Fold –
Pyramid – Child - Bridge – Corpse

HIP DISCOMFORT

HIP DISCOMFORT SEQUENCE ONE

This sequence is specifically for stiff hips and can also be used to prevent arthritis of the hips.

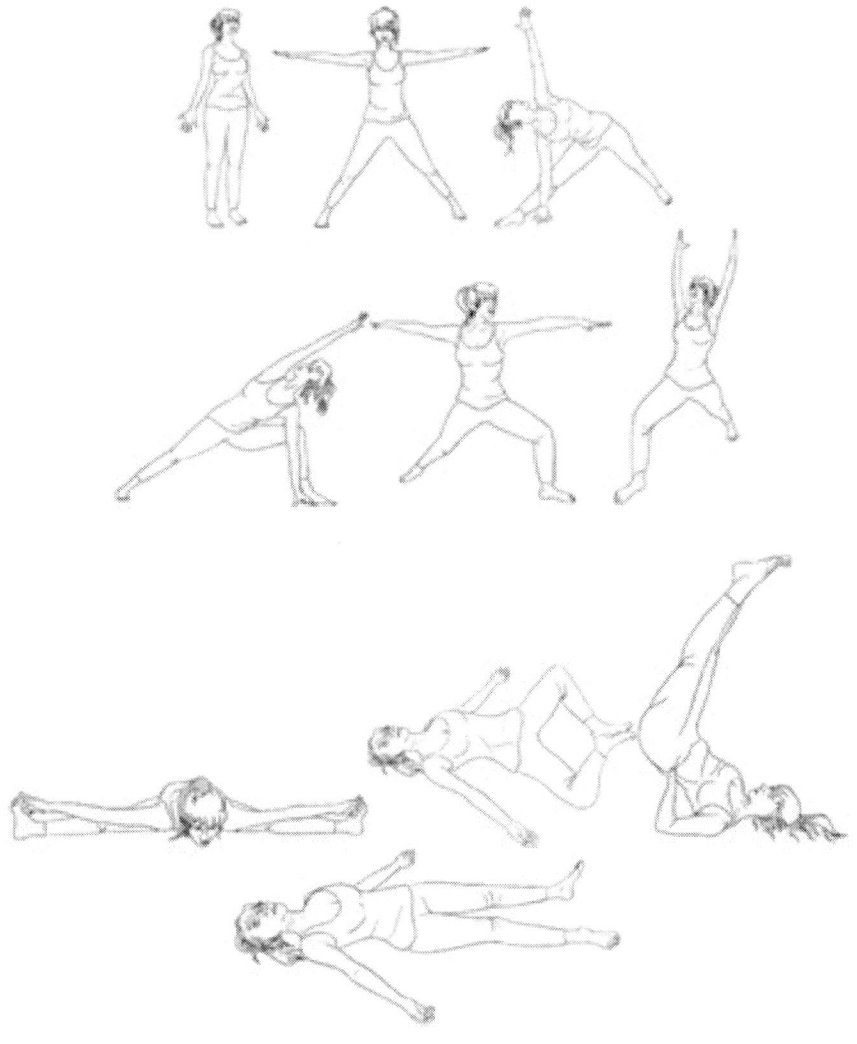

Mountain - Five Pointed Star – Triangle Extended Side Angle - Warrior Two -
Warrior One Seated Angle - Supine Bound Angle - Half Shoulder-stand - Corpse

HIP DISCOMFORT SEQUENCE TWO

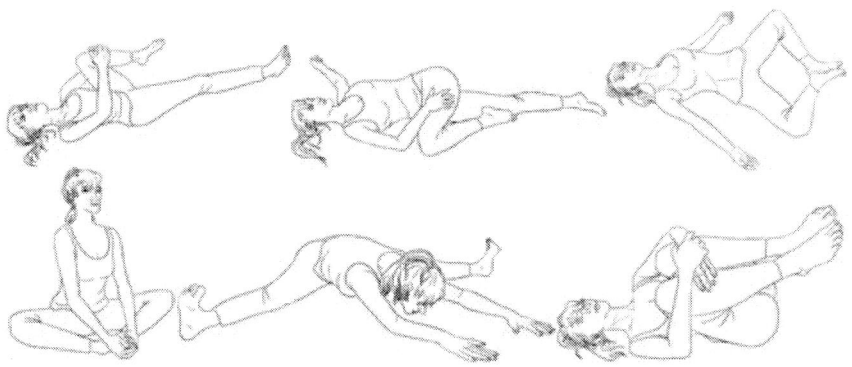

Half Wind Relieving - Knee Down Twist - Supine Bound Angel - Bound Angle -
Seated Angle – Wind Relieving

IMMUNITY

Also see the sequences for allergies, and cold & flu.

IMMUNITY SEQUENCE ONE

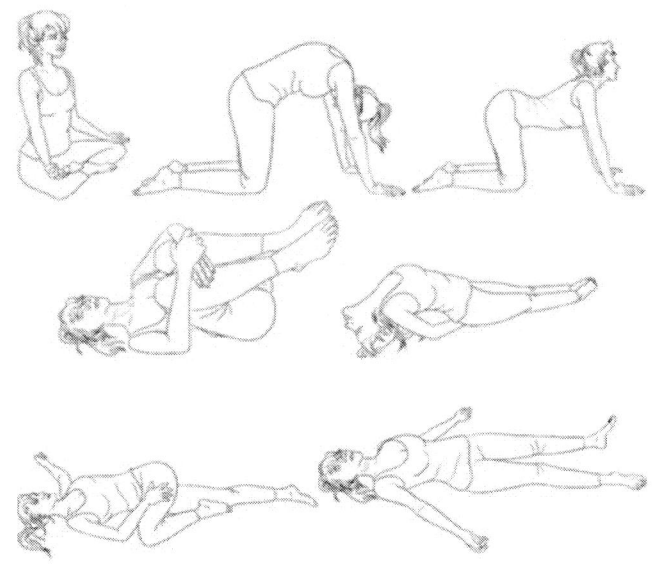

IMMUNITY SEQUENCE TWO

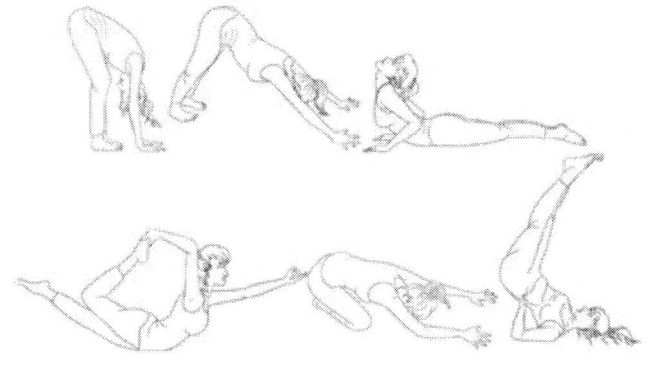

Standing Forward Fold - Downward Dog – Cobra - Half Bow –
Child - Half Shoulderstand

INDIGESTION

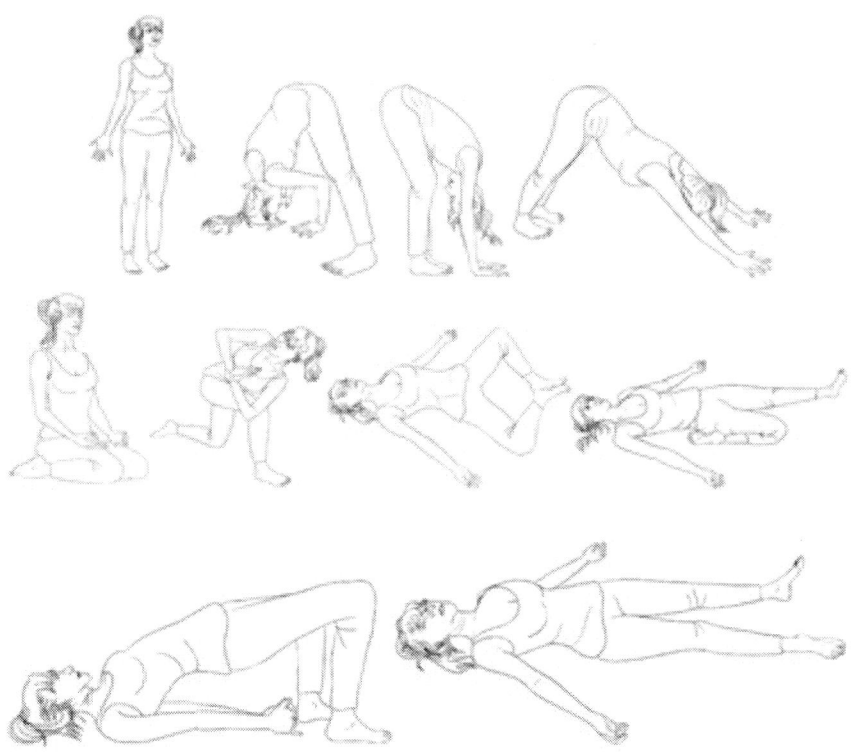

Mountain – Wide Legged Forward Bend - Standing Forward Fold - Downward Dog - Hero – Child - Half Prayer Twist - Supine Bound Angle - Half Supine Hero - Bridge – Corpse

INSOMNIA

Do these routines before going to bed.

INSOMNIA SEQUENCE ONE

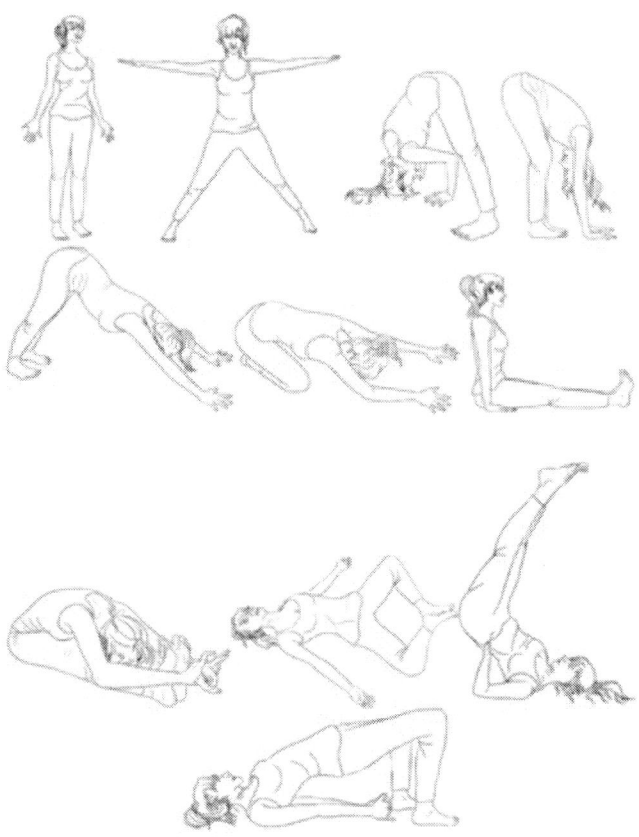

*Mountain - Five Pointed Star – Wide Legged Forward Bend -
Standing Forward Fold - Downward Dog – Child – Staff -
Seated Forward Bend - Supine Bound Angle - Half Shoulder-
stand - Bridge*

INSOMNIA SEQUENCE TWO

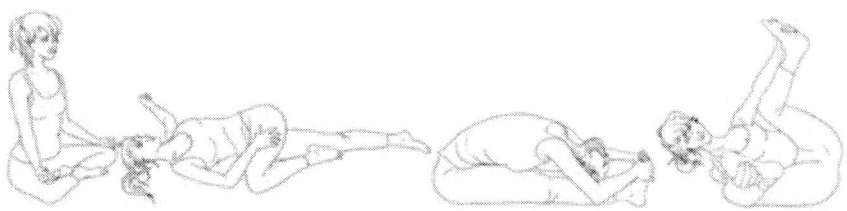

Accomplished (with meditation) - Knee Down Twist - Seated Forward Bend - Joyful Baby

KNEE PROBLEMS

When doing these sequences keep your legs strong and engaged. This will create space in the knee joint and also provides support.

Be careful not to do any jerking movements.

KNEE PROBLEMS SEQUENCE ONE

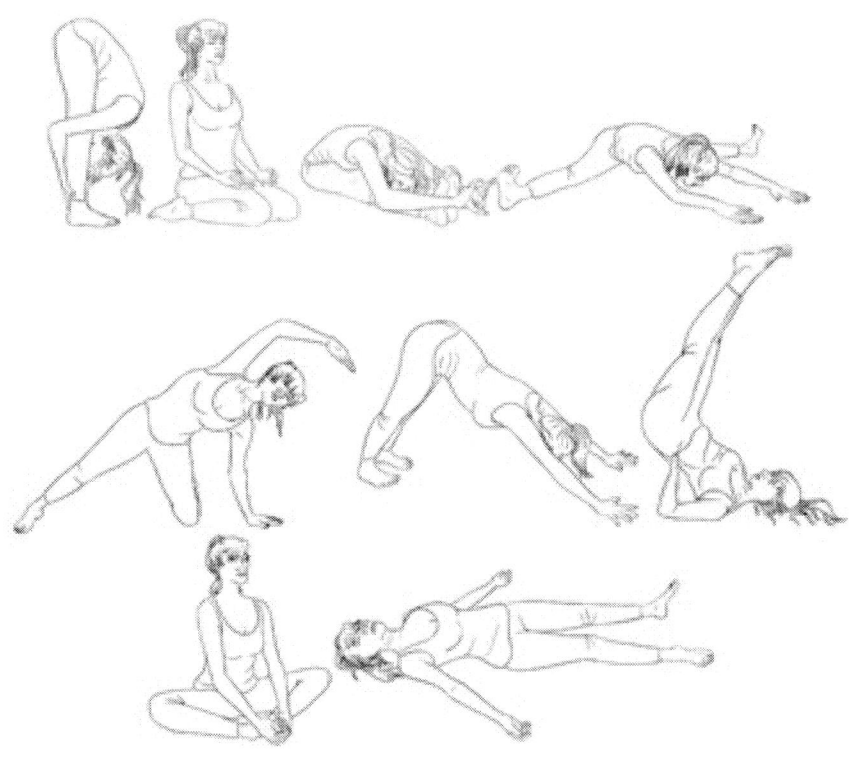

Standing Forward Fold – Hero - Seated Forward Bend – Seated Angle - Half Circle - Downward Dog - Half Shoulder-stand - Bound Angle – Corpse

KNEE PROBLEMS SEQUENCE TWO

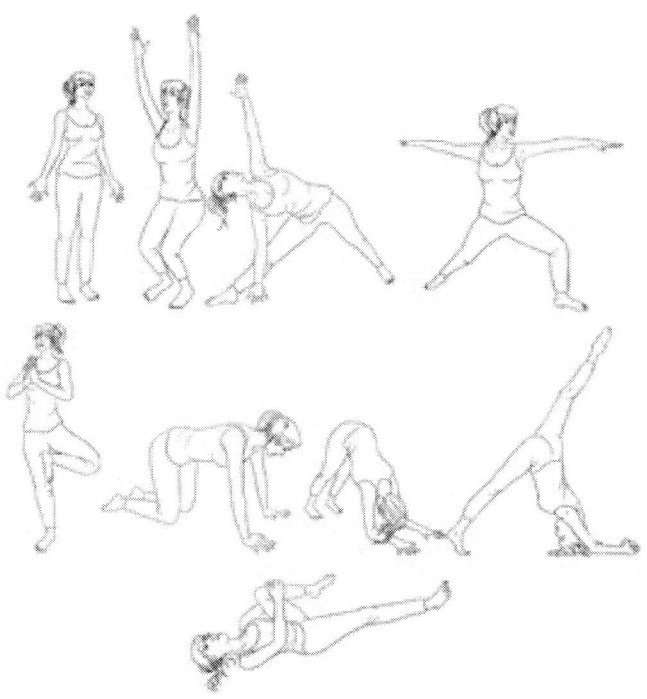

Mountain – Chair – Triangle - Warrior Two Tree – Table – Dolphin - One Legged Dolphin Half Wind Relieving

LETHARGY

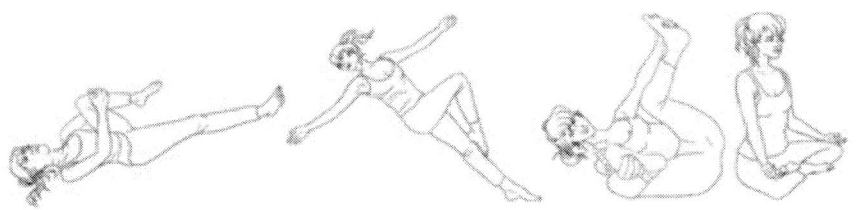

Half Wind Relieving - Knee Down Twist - Joyful Baby – Accomplished

LONG TRAVEL

You can use these routines any time you have been sitting for a long time.

LONG TRAVEL SEQUENCE ONE

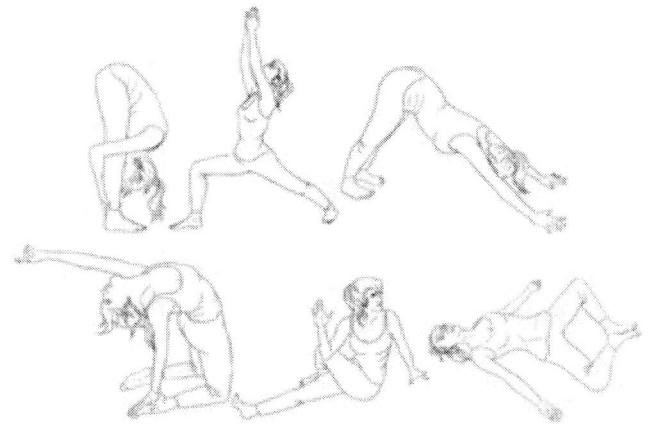

Standing Forward Fold - Warrior One - Downward Dog - Half Camel - Seated Spinal Twist - Supine Bound Angel

LONG TRAVEL SEQUENCE TWO

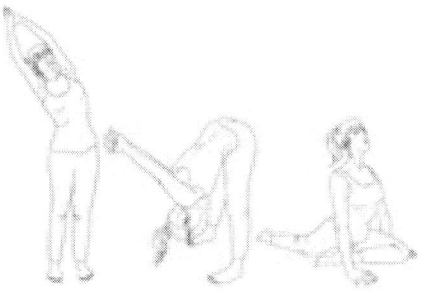

Crescent Moon - Standing Yoga Seal – Pigeon

LOW SELF-ESTEEM

LOW SELF-ESTEEM SEQUENCE ONE

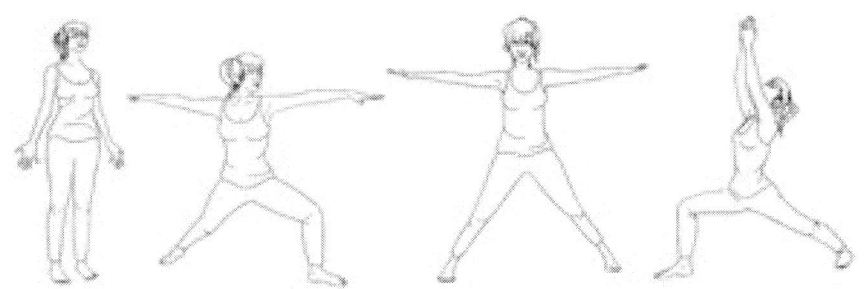

Mountain - Warrior Two - Five Pointed Star - Warrior One

LOW SELF-ESTEEM SEQUENCE TWO

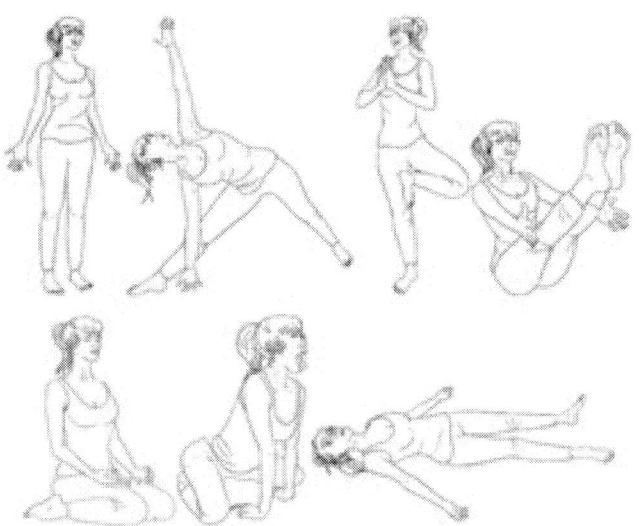

*Mountain – Triangle – Tree - Upward Boat - Hero – Lion -
Corpse (with yoga nidra)*

LOW SELF-ESTEEM SEQUENCE THREE

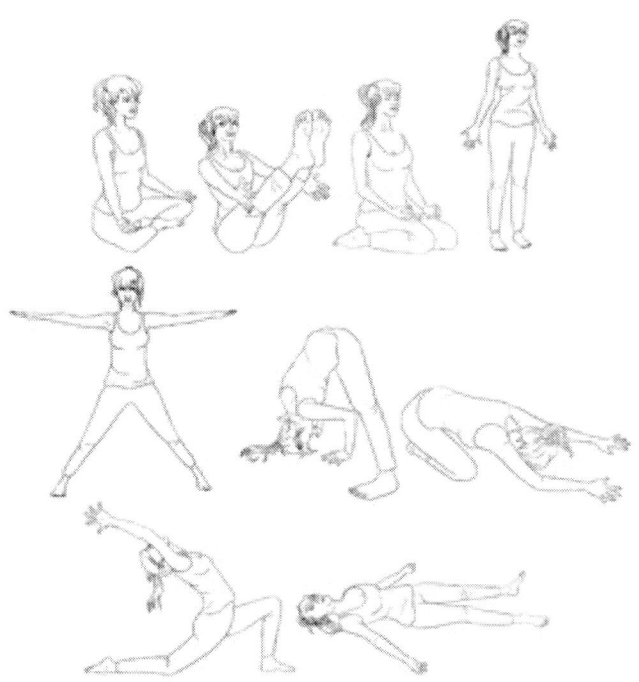

*Accomplished (with meditation) - Upward Boat - Hero –
Mountain - Five Pointed Star - Wide Legged Forward Bend –
Child - Low Warrior – Corpse (with yoga nidra)*

MENOPAUSE

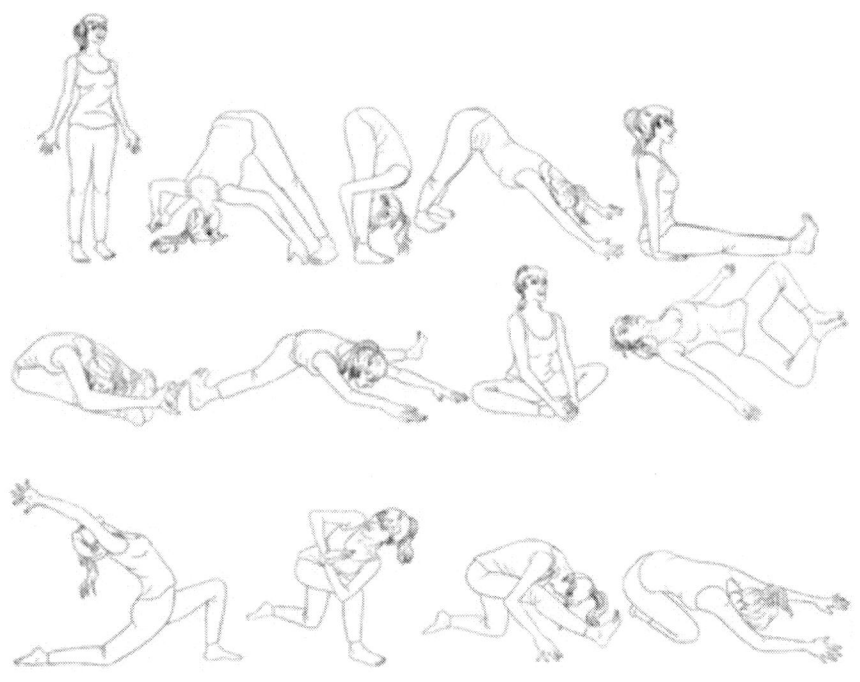

Mountain – Wide Legged Forward Bend - Standing Forward Fold - Downward Dog – Staff - Seated Forward Bend - Seated Angle - Bound Angle - Supine Bound Angle - Hero - Half Supine Hero - Half Shoulder-stand – Bridge - Corpse

HOT FLASHES

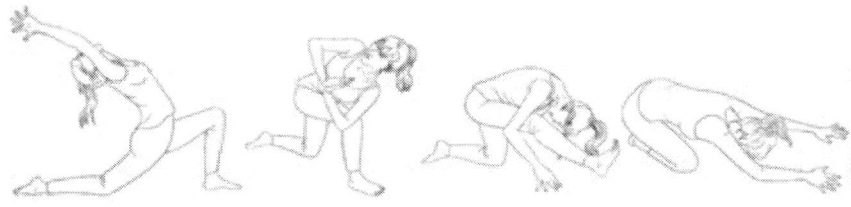

Low Warrior - Half Prayer Twist - Half Pyramid – Child

MENSTRUATION

The following sequences can give relief to discomforts you may feel during menstruation and if used regularly they can have permanent effects.

MENSTRUATION SEQUENCE ONE

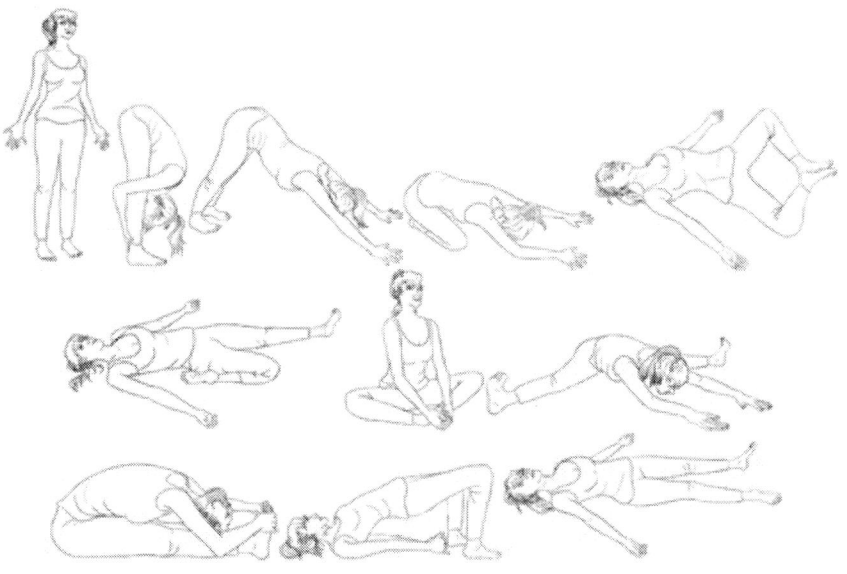

Mountain – Standing Forward Fold - Downward Dog – Child - Supine Bound Angle - Half Supine Hero - Bound Angle - Seated Angle - Seated Forward Bend – Bridge – Corpse

MENSTRUATION SEQUENCE TWO

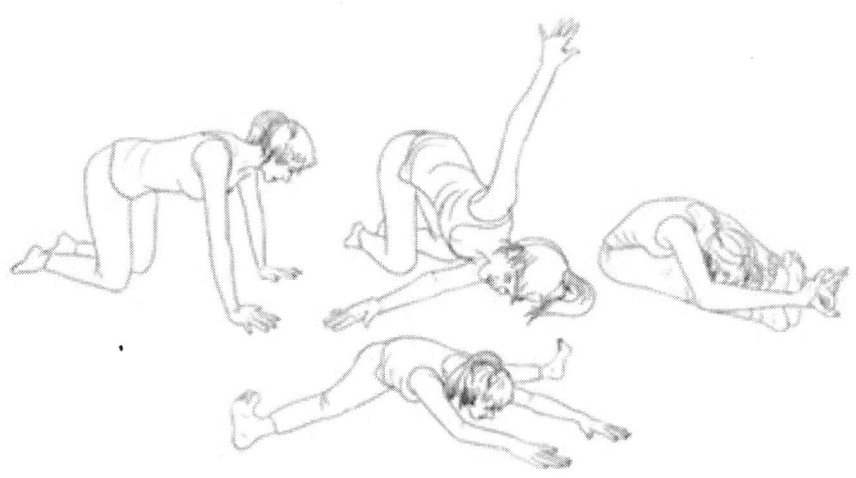

Table - Threading the Needle - Seated Forward Bend - Seated Angle

MENSTRUATION SEQUENCE THREE

This sequence is particularly useful for relieving menstrual cramps.

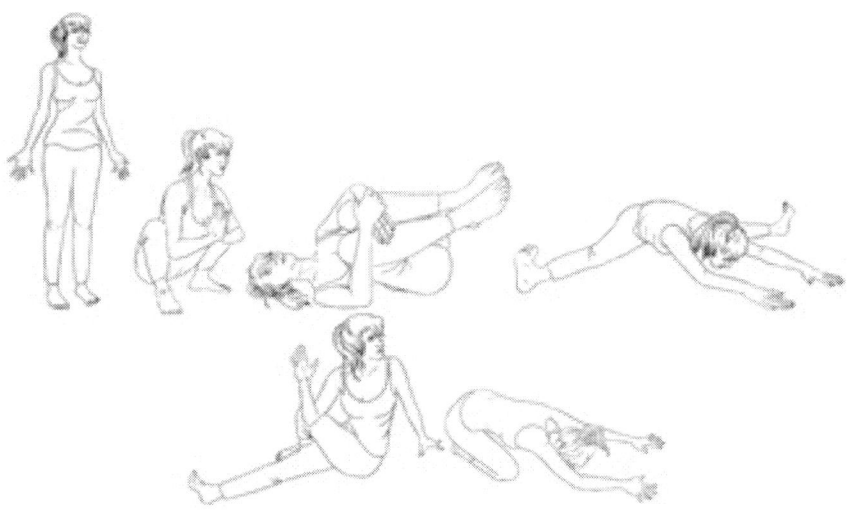

Mountain - Prayer Squat – Wind Relieving - Seated Angle Seated Spinal Twist –
Child

POSTURE

In order to correct your posture, you need to do the following routine regularly. Concentrate on having an open chest with your shoulders down and back.

POSTURE SEQUENCE ONE

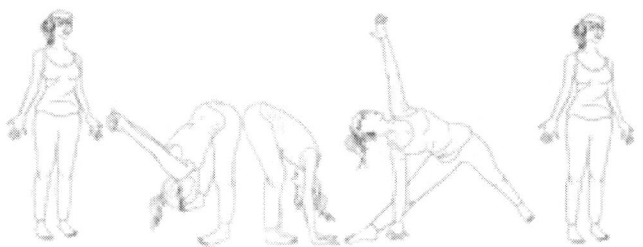

Mountain - Standing Yoga Seal - Standing Forward Fold –
Triangle – Mountain

POSTURE SEQUENCE TWO

This sequence focuses more on spinal alignment and flexibility.

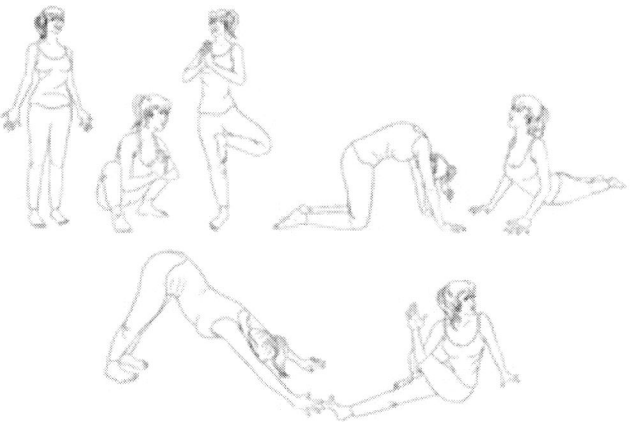

Mountain - Prayer Squat – Tree – Cat Tilt – Cobra - Downward
Dog - Seated Spinal Twist

PREGNANCY

Care must be taken when doing any physical activity during pregnancy and it is no different for yoga.

Do not do twists, especially during your first trimester, and it is best to avoid inversions (headstands, handstands, etc.)

It is highly recommended to seek advice from a professional yoga instructor as well as your doctor to discover the best way to continue your yoga practice while pregnant.

These two gentle routines can be done in any phase of pregnancy.

PREGNANCY SEQUENCE ONE

After completing this routine go for a walk.

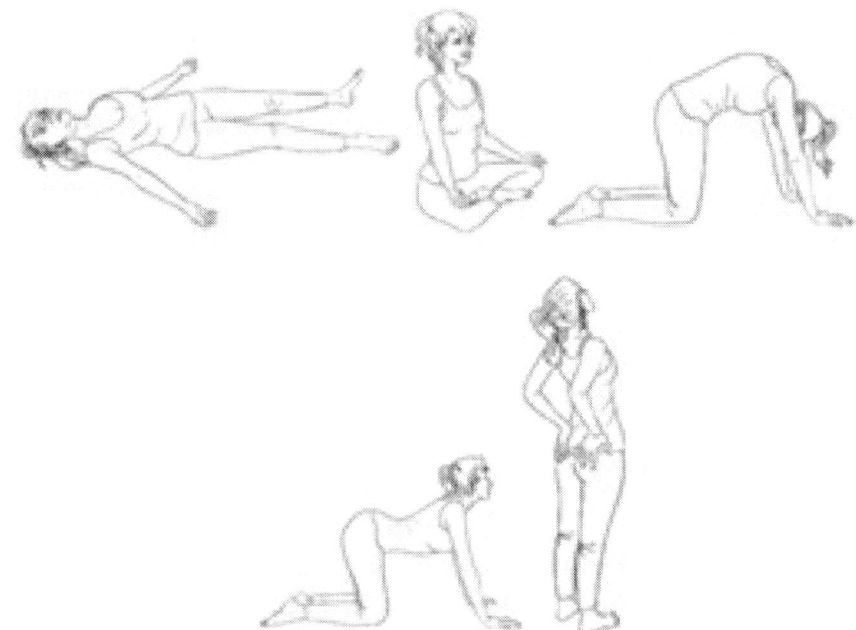

Corpse (with meditation) – Accomplished - Cat Tilt Dog Tilt – Standing Back Bend

PREGNANCY SEQUENCE TWO

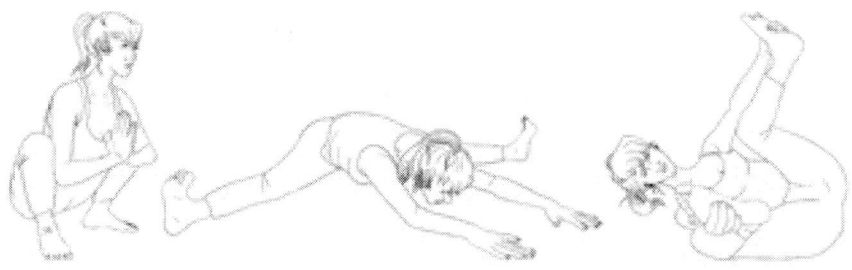

Prayer Squat - Seated Angle - Joyful Baby

PROCRASTINATION

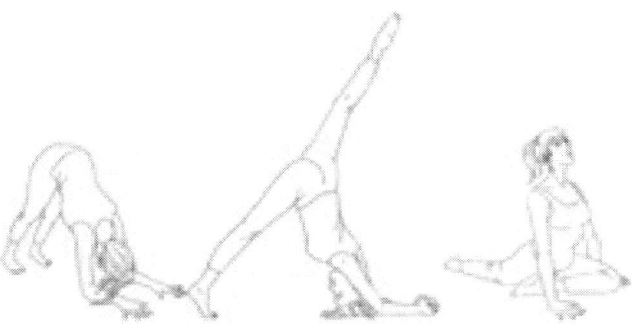

Dolphin - One Legged Dolphin – Pigeon

PROLAPSED UTERUS

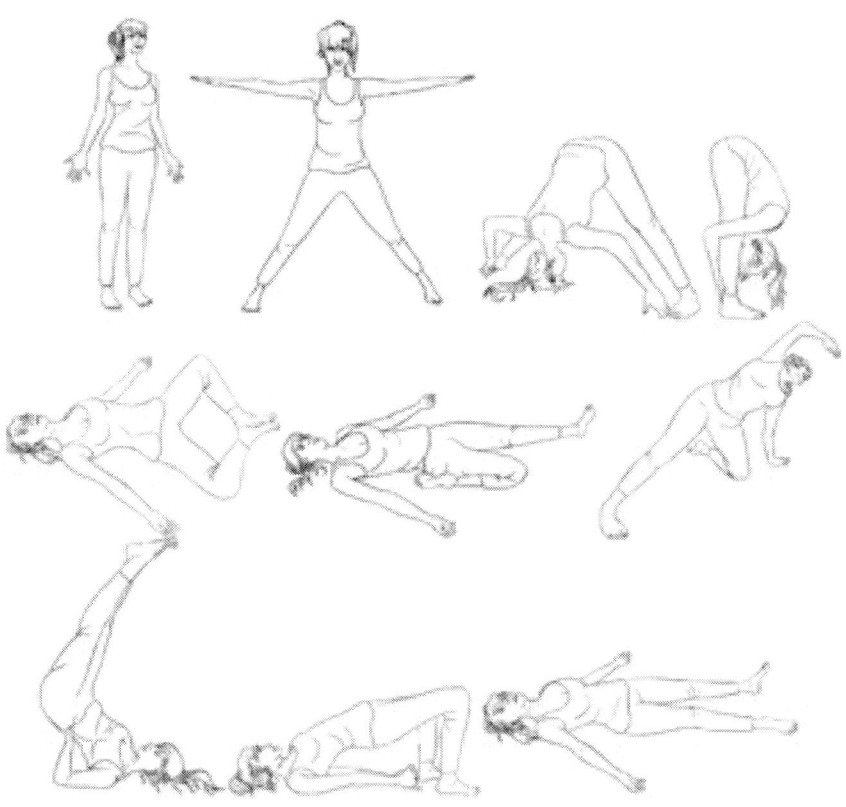

Mountain - Five Pointed Star – Wide Legged Forward Bend – Standing Forward Fold - Supine Bound Angle - Half Supine Hero – Half Circle - Half Shoulder-stand - Bridge – Corpse

RESPIRATORY AILMENTS

While doing this sequence pay special attention to opening your chest.

Practice this routine as well as the one for asthma and colds to increase strength in your respiratory system.

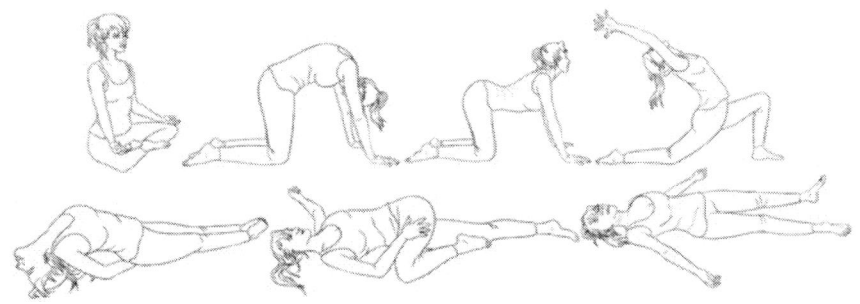

Accomplished (with alternating nostril breathing) - Cat Tilt - Dog Tilt - Low Warrior - Fish - Knee Down Twist – Corpse

RUNNER'S ACHES

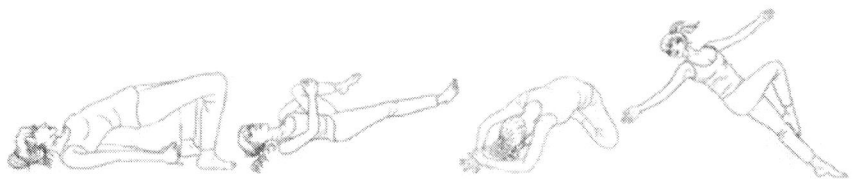

Bridge - Half Wind Relieving - Seated Head to Knee - Knee Down Twist

SHIN SPLINTS

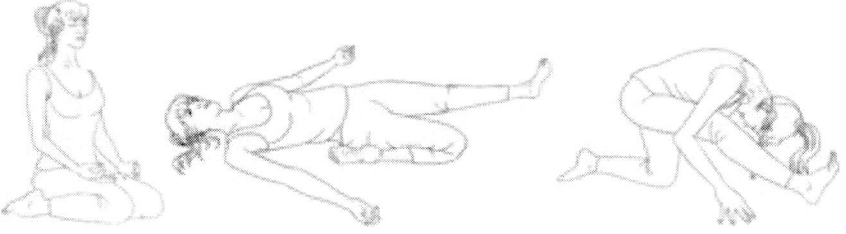

Hero - Half Supine Hero - Half Pyramid

SCIATICA

SCIATICA SEQUENCE ONE

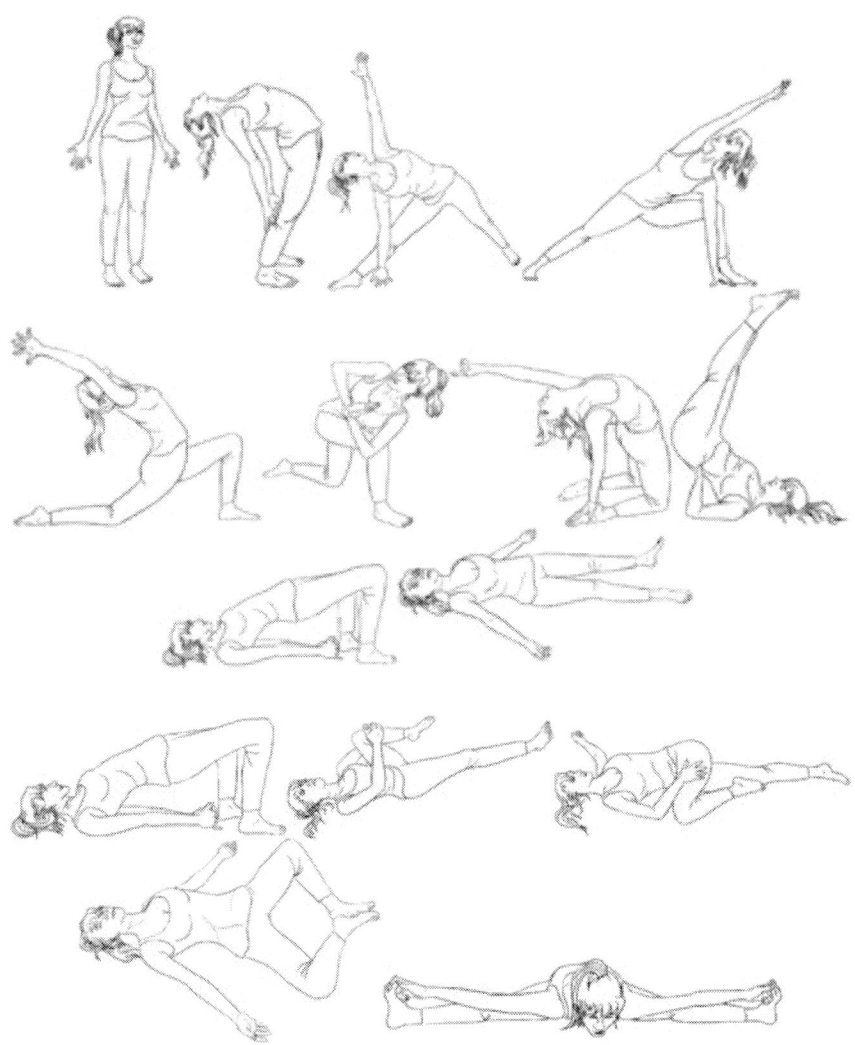

Mountain - Standing Back Bend - Triangle - Extended Side Angle - Low Warrior -
Half Prayer Twist - Half Camel - Half Shoulder-stand - Bridge – Corpse

SCIATICA SEQUENCE TWO

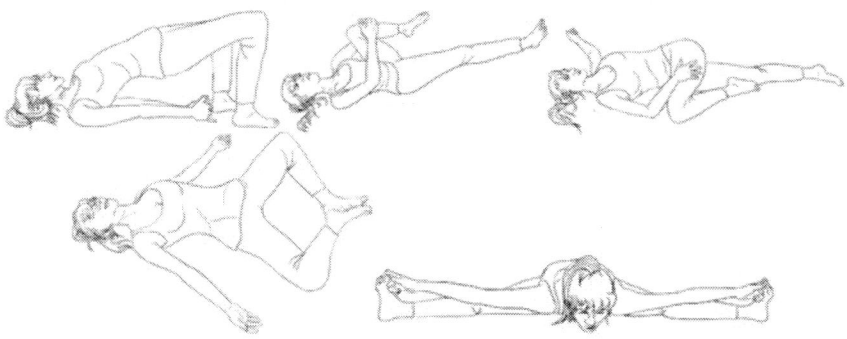

Bridge - Half Wind Relieving - Knee Down Twist - Supine Bound Angle - Seated Angle

STOMACH PROBLEMS

STOMACH ACHE

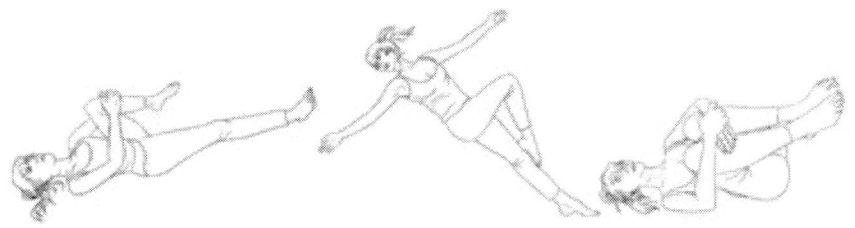

Half Wind Relieving - Knee Down Twist - Wind Relieving

DIGESTION

This sequence will strengthen your digestive system.

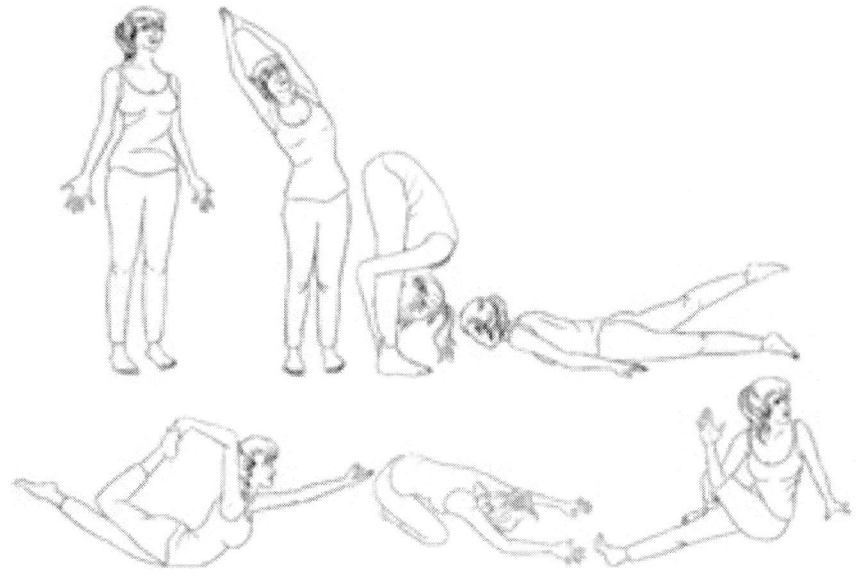

*Mountain - Crescent Moon – Standing Forward Fold - Half Locust - Half Bow –
Child - Seated Spinal Twist*

CONSTIPATION

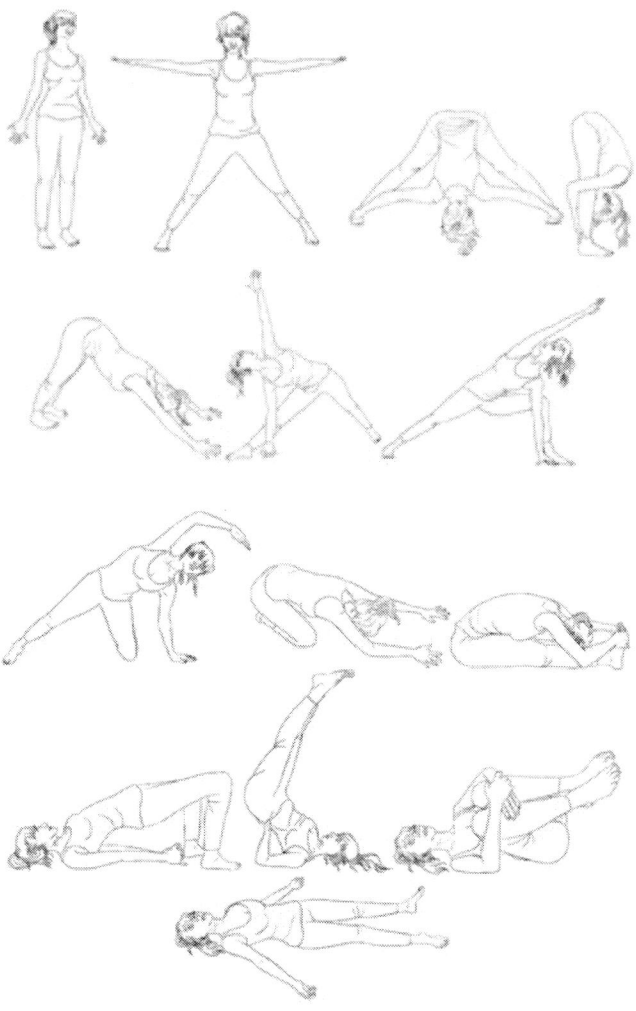

*Mountain - Five Pointed Star – Wide Legged Forward Bend -
Standing Forward Fold - Downward Dog - Triangle - Extended
Side Angle - Half Circle – Child - Seated Forward Bend - Bridge -
Half Shoulder-stand – Wind Relieving - Corpse*

DIARRHEA

Ensure that your abdomen is not cramped or restricted whilst doing this sequence.

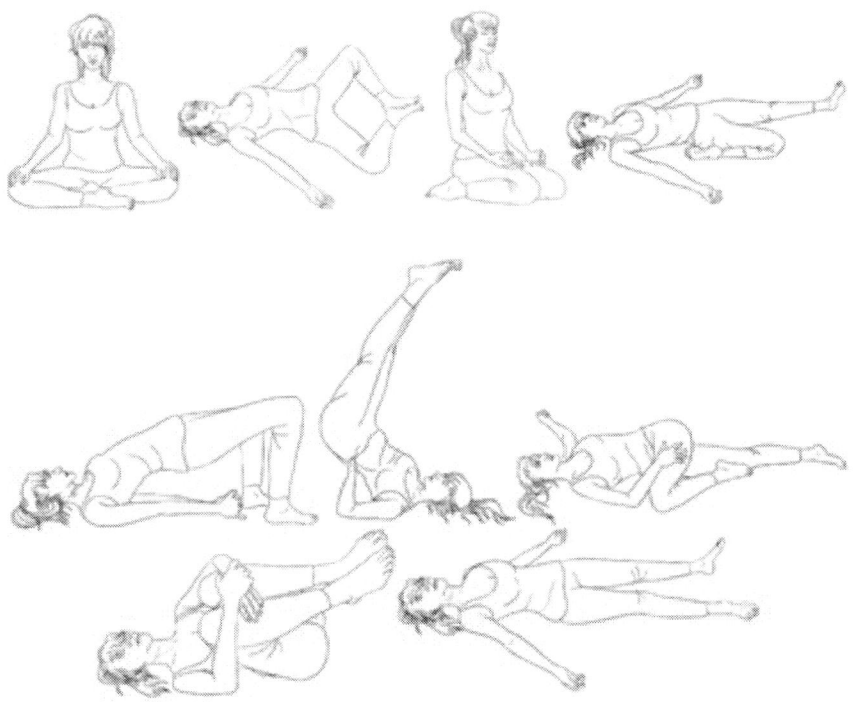

Accomplished - Supine Bound Angle – Hero - Half Supine Hero - Bridge - Half Shoulder-stand - Knee Down Twist - Wind Relieving – Corpse

STRENGTH

This sequence is good for all over body strength.

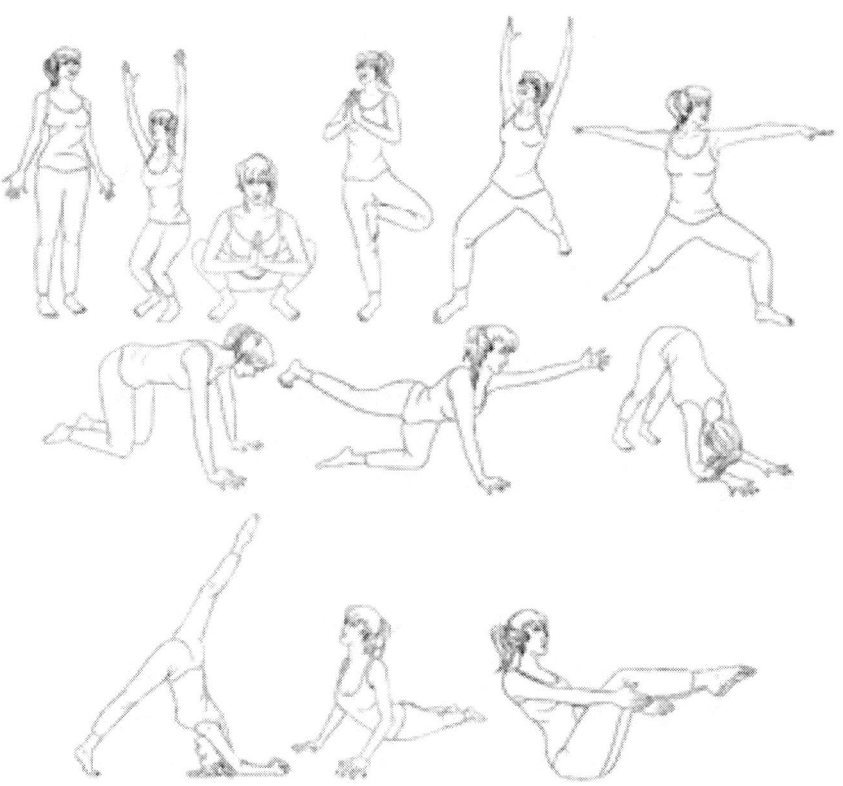

Mountain – Chair - Prayer Squat – Tree - Warrior One - Warrior Two - Table –
Balancing Table – Dolphin One Legged Dolphin – Cobra – Upward Boat

STRESS AND ANXIETY

Regular practice of these sequences has a long lasting effect on lowering stress and anxiety.

Keep your whole face relaxed.

STRESS AND ANXIETY SEQUENCE ONE

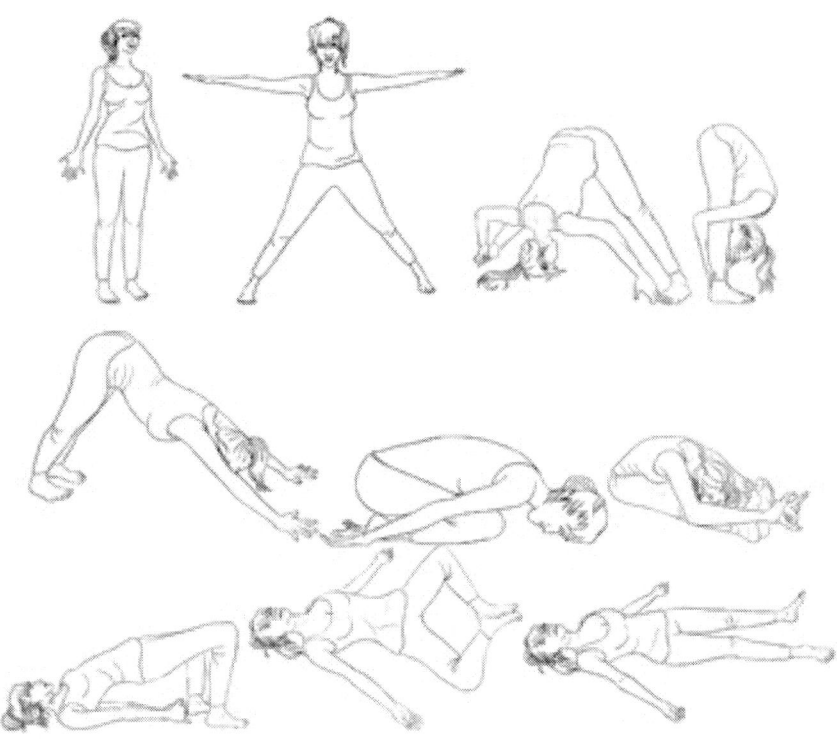

Mountain - Five Pointed Star – Wide Legged Forward Bend - Standing Forward Fold - Downward Dog – Child - Seated Forward Bend - Bridge - Supine Bound Angle – Corpse (with yoga nidra)

STRESS AND ANXIETY SEQUENCE TWO

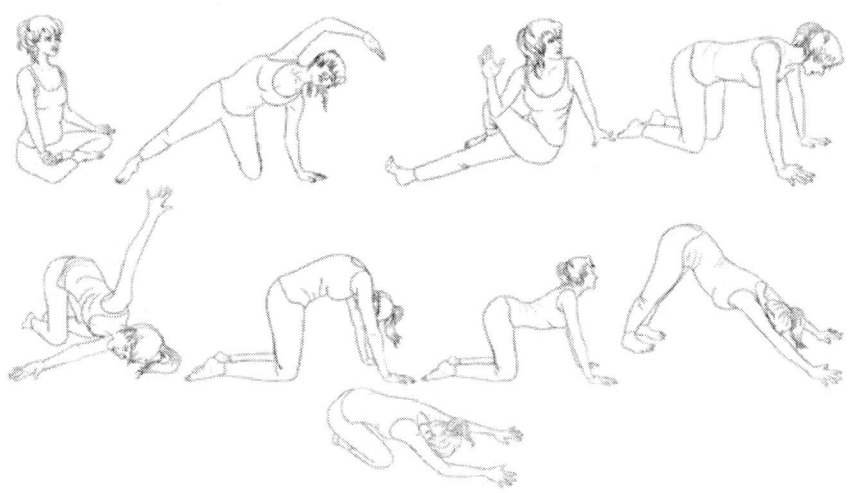

Accomplished (with alternate nostril breathing) - Half Circle - Seated Spinal Twist – Table - Threading the Needle – Cat Tilt – Dog Tilt - Downward Dog - Child (with meditation)

STRESS AND ANXIETY SEQUENCE THREE

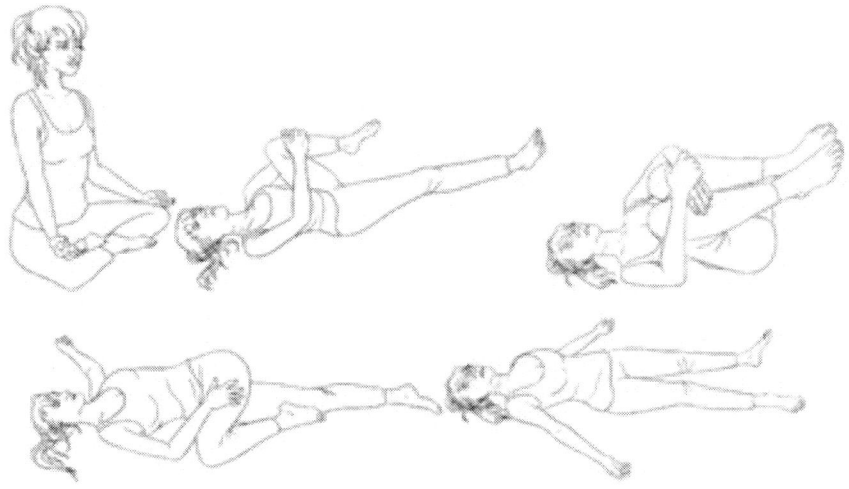

Accomplished (with meditation) – Half Wind Relieving - Wind Relieving - Knee Down Twist – Corpse

STRESS AND ANXIETY SEQUENCE FOUR

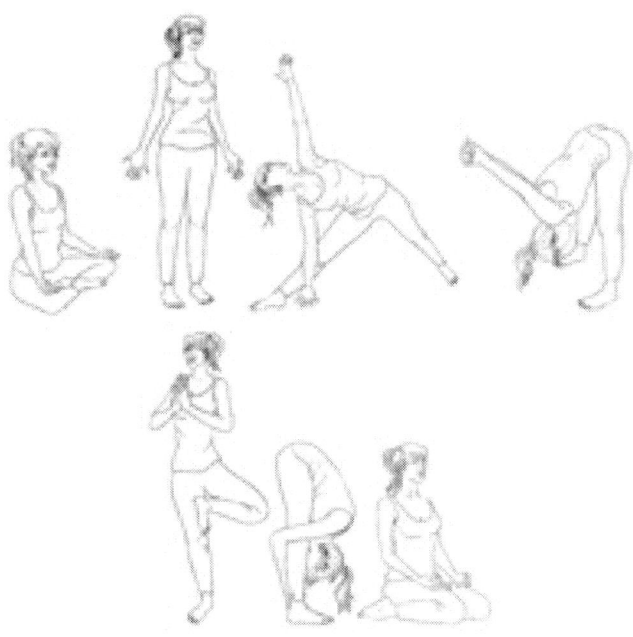

*Accomplished (with meditation) – Mountain – Triangle -
Standing Yoga Seal - Tree – Standing Forward Fold - Hero (with
meditation)*

TENSE SHOULDERS AND NECK

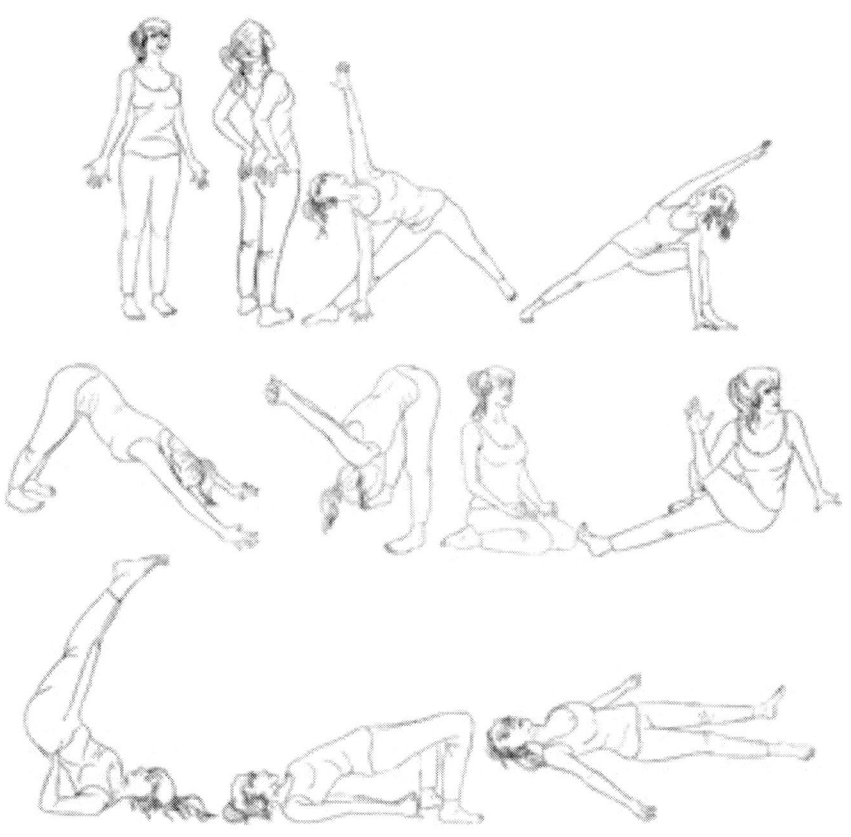

Mountain - Standing Backbend – Triangle - Extended Side Angle - Downward Dog – Standing Yoga Seal – Hero – Seated Spinal Twist - Half Shoulder-stand – Bridge – Corpse

THYROID IMBALANCE

This short routine is aimed at restoring overall balance to the thyroid.

Specific thyroid conditions need specific treatments. Use this sequence as a supplement to your health professionals advised treatment.

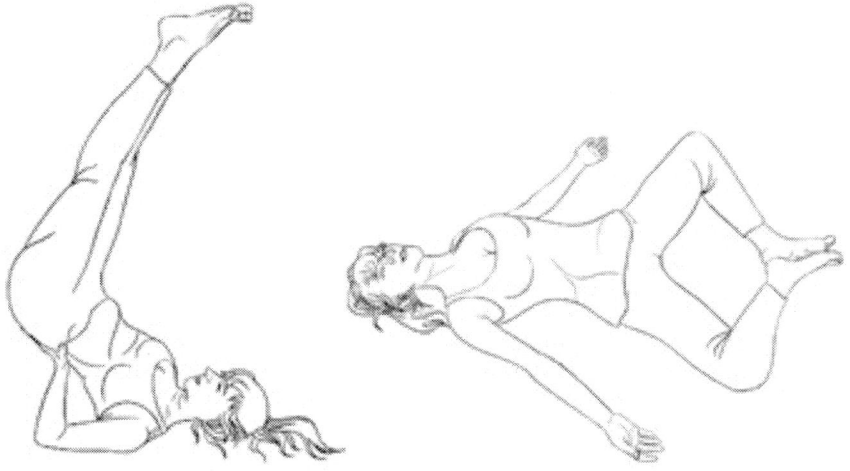

Half Shoulder Stand - Supine Bound Angle

TOXIN FLUSH

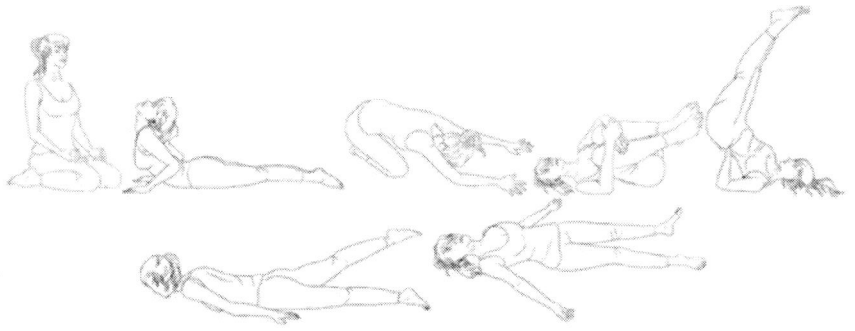

Hero – Cobra – Child – Wind Relieving - Half Shoulder-stand - Half Locust - Corpse (with Yoga Nidra)

VARICOSE VEINS

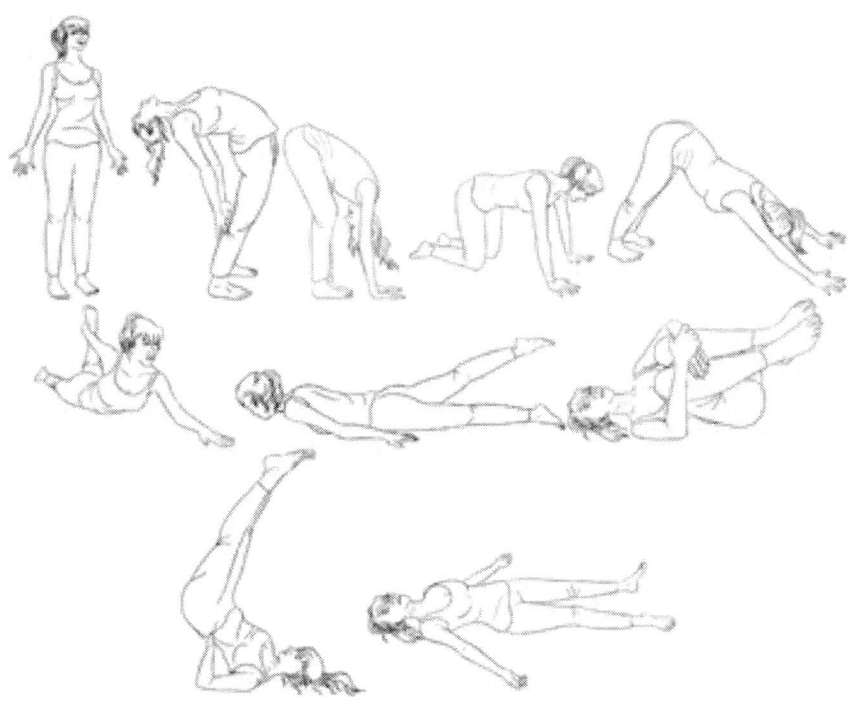

Mountain – Standing Back Bend – Standing Forward Fold – Table - Downward Dog - Half Bow - Half Locust – Wind Relieving - Half Shouldestand – Corpse

VERTIGO / DIZZY SPELL

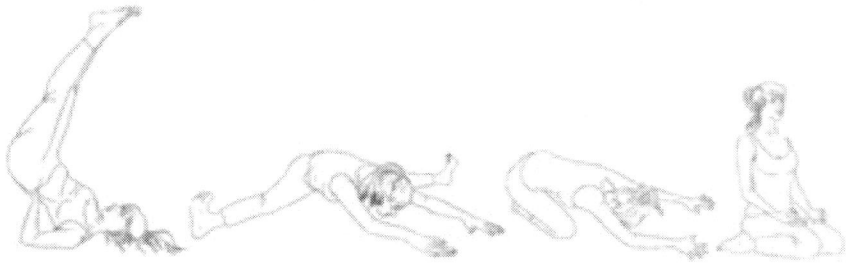

Half Shoulder-stand - Seated Angle – Child - Hero (with meditation)

POSES

Although all the poses used in this book are considered to be of a basic level, when first starting you may find some of them challenging.

Adjust them to your comfort level and work your way up. Hold each pose where you can feel a good stretch but not pain.

You will probably notice your breath shorten if you try to force your body too much. When this happens just back of a little and re-focus on your breathing.

If you do find yourself in a painful position, back out of it slowly to avoid injury.

ACCOMPLISHED POSE

Avoid if you have a hip, and/or knee injury.

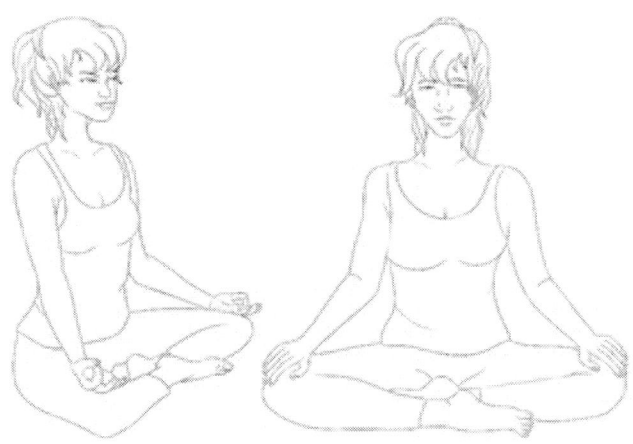

Sit with your buttocks on the floor, legs crossed.

Have both heels close to your midline by putting one foot near your inner thigh and the other one near your ankle.

Rest your hands in your lap or on your knees. Your palms can face either up, down, or in a mudra.

Lengthen your spine by stretching the crown of your head towards the sky as you press your hips down.

Push your chest forward and drop your shoulders. Relax your whole face and belly.

BALANCING TABLE

Avoid if you have an arm, back, knee, and/or shoulder injury.

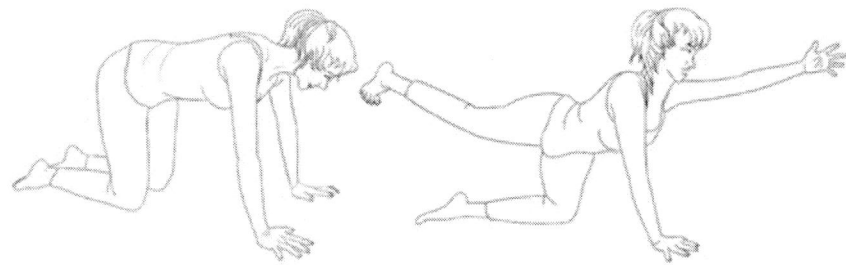

Starting in table pose, as you inhale, lift your right leg so it is parallel to the ground with your toes pointing behind you.

Raise your left arm so it is also parallel to the ground with your fingers pointing in front of you.

When you are ready exhale as you bring your arm down first and then your knee back into table.

BOUND ANGLE

Avoid if you have a hip and/or knee injury.

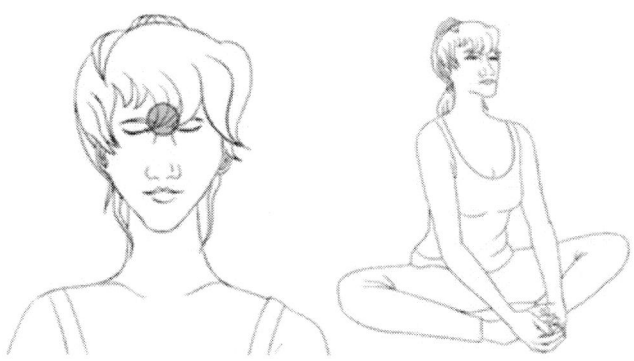

Start in staff pose.

Bend your legs to bring the bottoms of your feet together. Your knees bend facing out. Hold onto your toes by interlacing your fingers around them.

As you inhale stretch the crown of your head up towards the sky while pushing your hips down. Push your chest forward and relax your shoulders down.

Close your eyes and look to your third eye (behind the middle of your forehead). As you exhale push your knees to the ground and gently pull your torso forward. Ensure to keep your chest open and back flat.

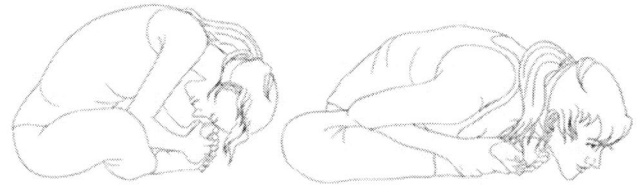

For a deeper stretch, pull your forehead or chest towards your feet. When you're ready, return to staff pose.

CORPSE POSE

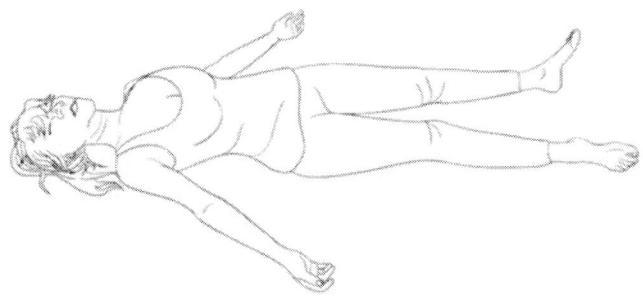

Lie flat on your back on the floor. You can place a pillow under your head if you want.

Keep your head straight, i.e., don't let it fall to the side.

Draw your shoulder blades down and open your chest towards your chin.

Have your arms at a comfortable distance from your body with your palms facing up. Completely relax your arms and fingers.

Lift and extend your buttocks to your heels so that your whole sacrum rests on the floor.

Keep your abdomen soft and relaxed.

Slowly stretch your legs out straight one at the time. Allow them to roll out to the side from the hips to the feet. Check that your body is in a straight line and you are resting evenly on the left and right sides.

Once you are comfortable stay perfectly still and quiet and be aware of your body relaxing deeper into the floor.

Allow your eyes to rest completely so they sink deeper towards the back of the skull. Relax your whole face and body.

Be aware of your breath, quiet and soft.

BRIDGE POSE

Avoid if you have a back, knee, and/or shoulder injury.

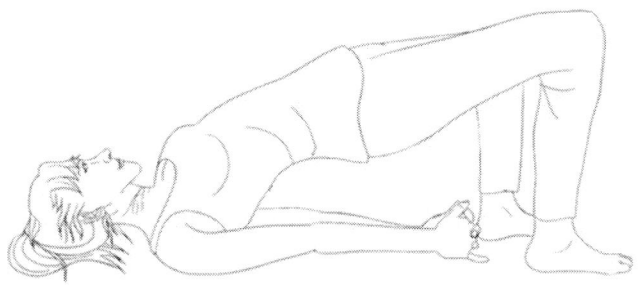

Lie down on your back and bend your knees up so that your feet are flat on the floor, hip width apart.

Place your arms on the ground, straight but relaxed, palms down with your finger-tips just touching your heels.

As you inhale push your feet into the ground and lift your hips up so that your spine rolls off the floor. Keep your knees hip-width apart.

Interlace your fingers underneath your back and lift your chest by pressing your arms and shoulders down. Use your buttocks, legs, and perineum muscles to lift your hips higher.

When you're ready, exhale and slowly roll your spine back to the ground.

CATERPILLAR POSE

Avoid if you have a back, elbow, neck, shoulder, and/or wrist injury.

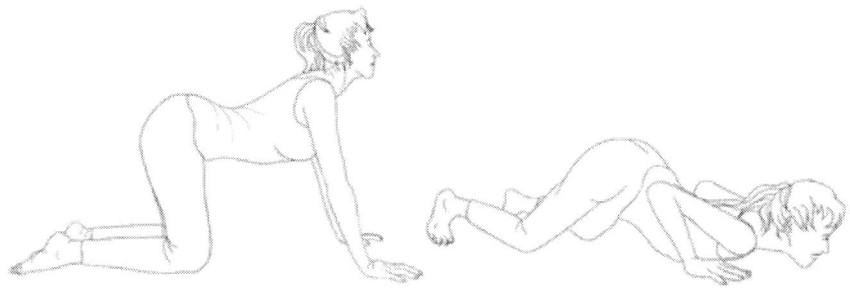

Adopt dog tilt and then lower your chest and chin to the ground as you exhale. Your chest is between your palms.

Push your chest to the ground as you raise your tailbone to the sky. Keep your elbows close to your sides.

You can inhale into dog tilt and exhale into eight limbed and number of times.

CAT TILT
Avoid if you have a back injury.

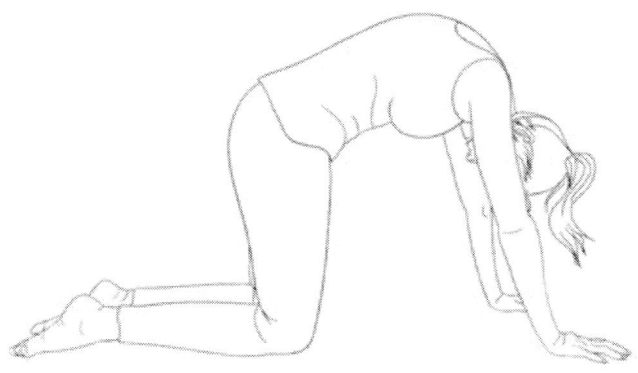

Start in table pose.

As you exhale let your head and shoulders drop down and round your spine towards the sky.

You can inhale into dog tilt and exhale into cat tilt a couple of times before settling back into table pose.

CHAIR POSE

Avoid if you have a back, hip, knee, and/or shoulder injury.

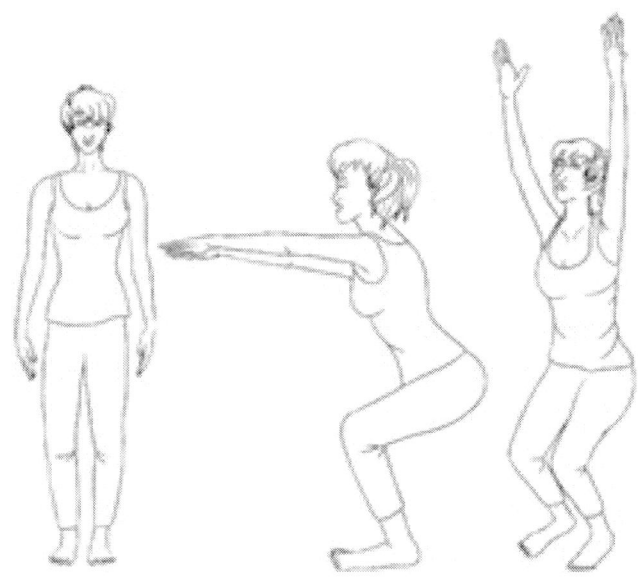

Starting in mountain pose, as you inhale raise your arms forward so they are parallel to the ground.

Squat down at your knees as you breathe out. Have your knees pointing forward and shift your weight to your heels as you move your hips down and back.

Ensure your hips do not sink below your knees. Pretend you are sitting on the edge of a chair.

Arch your spine by pressing your shoulders down and back. Relax your shoulders and stretch out through your fingertips.

For more of a challenge raise your arms to the sky and look up.

When ready inhale as you straighten your legs and raise your arms to the sky, then exhale and lower your arms back into mountain.

CHILD POSE

Avoid if you have a knee injury.

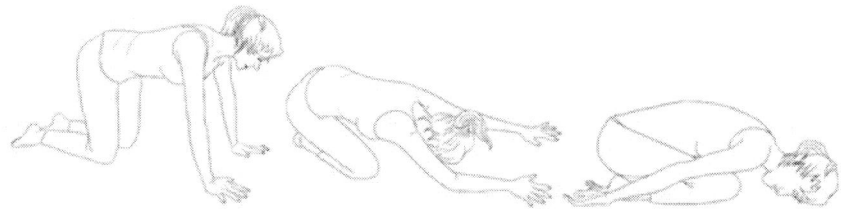

Starting in table pose, as you exhale lower your hips to your heels and then place your forehead on the ground with your arms in front of you, palms face down.

You can also put your arms down along the sides of your body with your palms facing up. Your knees can be together or slightly apart.

Press your belly against your thighs as you inhale.

When you are ready place your palms under your shoulders and inhale as you come up to a seated position.

COBRA POSE

Avoid if you have an arm, back, and/or shoulder injury, and/or have had recent abdominal surgery, and/or are pregnant.

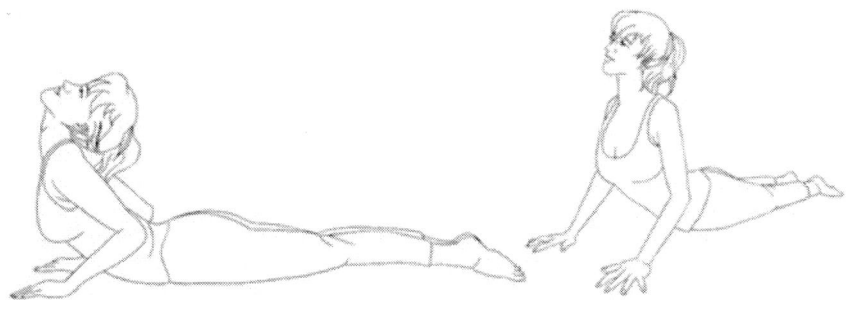

Lie on your stomach with your chin on the ground and your legs together.

Place your palms flat on the ground under your shoulders, elbows close to your sides.

Press your pubic bone into the ground and engage your buttocks, kneecaps, perineum, and thighs.

As you inhale, without using your arms, lift your head and chest off the ground. Keep your neck and spine aligned.

Now press down into your palms to lift yourself higher.

Push your chest forward as you relax your shoulders back and down.

When ready lower your chest and head back to the ground as you exhale.

CRAB POSE

Avoid if you have an arm, back, hip, knee, and/or shoulder injury.

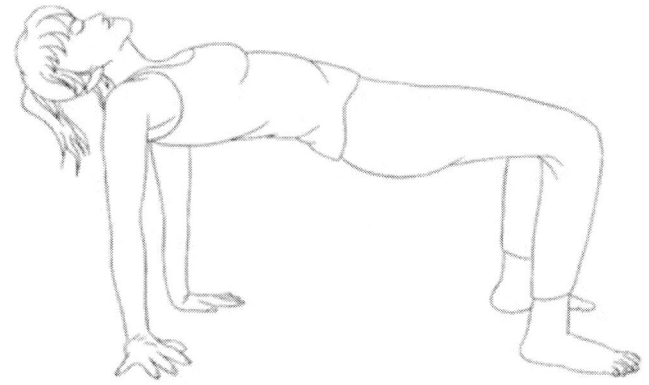

From staff pose place your hands behind your hips with your fingers facing forward. If you have wrist pain, you can make fists instead. Bend you knees up so that your feet are flat on the floor, hip width apart, with your knees and toes pointing forward.

As you inhale lean back into your arms and engage your whole body to lift your hips towards the sky. Look straight up to the sky or carefully allow your head to drop back.

When ready exhale as your lower your hips back to the ground.

CRESCENT MOON

Avoid if you have a back, hip, and/or shoulder injury.

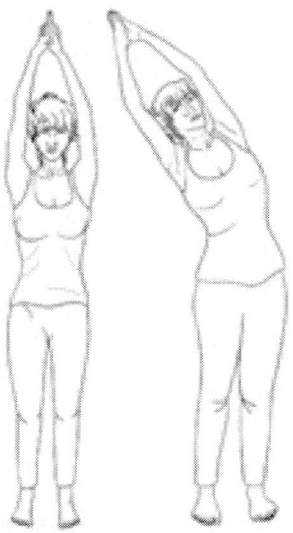

While inhaling adopt mountain pose with your fingers interlaced and your index fingers pointing to the sky.

As you exhale press your left hip out to the side and arch to your right.

Keep your body strong and lengthened.

Inhale as you return to the position with your fingers interlaced and your index fingers pointing to the sky.

Repeat it on your other side.

CROCODILE POSE

Avoid if pregnant.

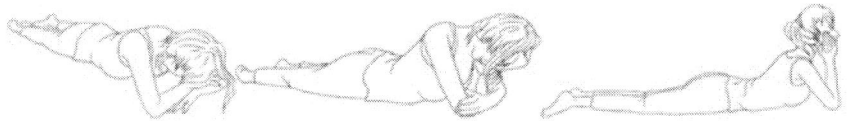

Lie on your stomach and cross your arms under your head, resting your forehead on your wrists.

Alternatively, lift your torso up by crossing your arms with your elbows under your shoulders and then allowing your head to hang, or, rest your chin in your palms with your elbows on the floor.

Allow your body to completely relax.

With each inhale press your belly into the ground. With each exhale relax your body deeper and deeper.

DOG TILT

Avoid if you have a back injury.

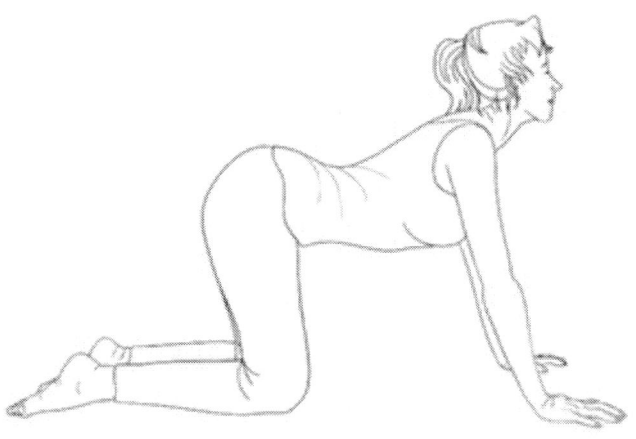

Begin in table pose.

As you inhale arch your spine by letting your belly drop down and reaching your tailbone towards the ceiling.

Press your palms into the ground as you spread your fingers wide apart. Drop your shoulders and you look up to the sky as high as you can without straining.

DOLPHIN POSE

Avoid if you have an arm, back, and/or shoulder injury, and/or have glaucoma, and/or unmediated high blood pressure.

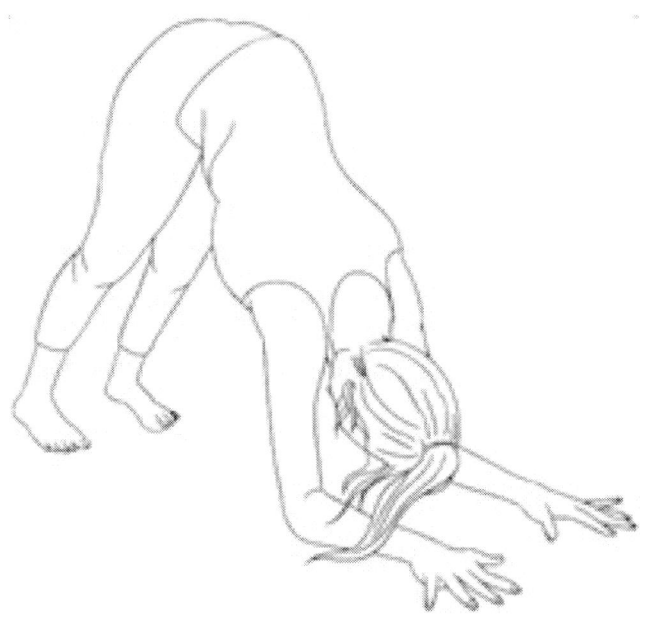

Starting in table pose get on the balls of your feet, lower your forearms to the ground, and lift your hips to the sky.

Ensure your palms and feet are shoulder width apart with your middle fingers and toes facing forwards. Spread your fingers as wide as you can.

Press into the floor with your hands and feet as you push your hips up and back. Ensure to keep your spine strong and lengthen it through your tailbone. Feel the stretch in the back of your legs. Keep your back straight. You can bend the back of your knees a little if you need to.

Let your head hang and rest your forehead on the floor.

DOWNWARD DOG

Avoid if you have an arm, back, hip, and/or shoulder injury, and/or unmediated high blood pressure.

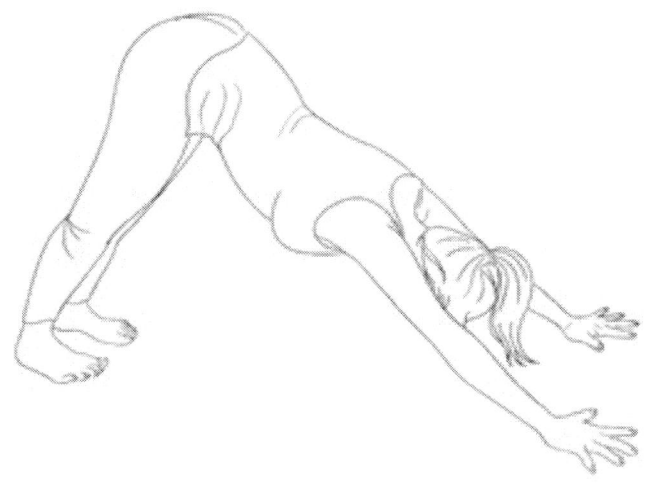

Start in table pose.

Inhale as you tuck your toes so you are on the balls of your feet. Keep your palms shoulder width apart and spread your fingers apart with your middle fingers facing forward.

Press into your hands and lift your hips towards the sky.

Push your hips up and back. Your chest goes towards your thighs. Have straight arms but do not lock your elbows.

Keep your spine straight as you lift up through your tailbone.

Stretch the back of your legs by pressing your heels to the floor. Keep your back flat. Your legs are straight (knees not locked) or with a small bend at the knees.

Let your head dangle freely.

DOWNWARD FACING FROG

Avoid if you have a knee, hip, and/or leg injury.

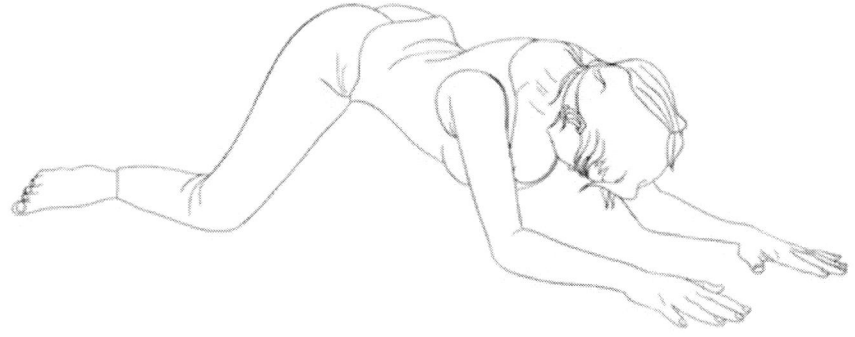

From hero pose, spread your knees as wide as you comfortably can and align your feet so that they are directly behind them, i.e. right foot behind right knee and left foot behind left knee.

Turn your feet outwards so your toes are facing away from your body.

Place your elbows, forearms, and palms flat on the floor.

Exhale as you push your hips back.

When ready bring your hips forward and place your palms under your shoulders to adopt table pose.

EXTENDED DOG

Avoid if you have an arm, back, knee, and/or shoulder injury.

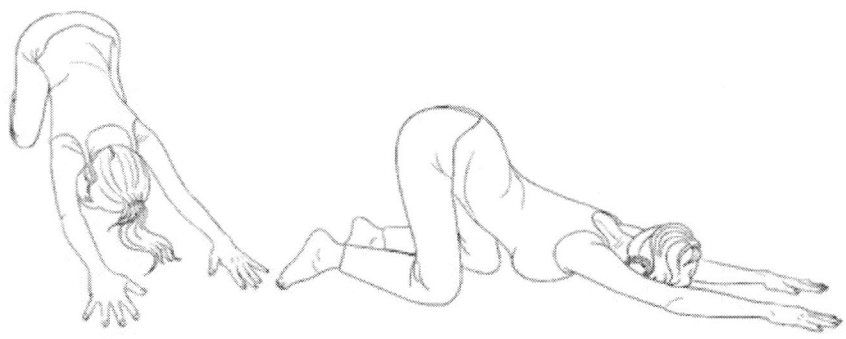

Start in table pose.

As you inhale push your tailbone towards the sky then exhale and lower your forehead to the floor by sliding your hands forward. Ensure you keep your hips lifted over your knees.

Arch the middle of your back by allowing your chest to sink towards the floor.

Deepen the stretch by straightening your arms, lifting your elbows off the floor, and bringing your hips back. Try not to let your hands slide while you do this.

Place your chin on the ground to stretch your neck.

When ready inhale and return to the table pose.

EXTENDED PIGEON

Avoid if you have a back, hip, and/or knee injury.

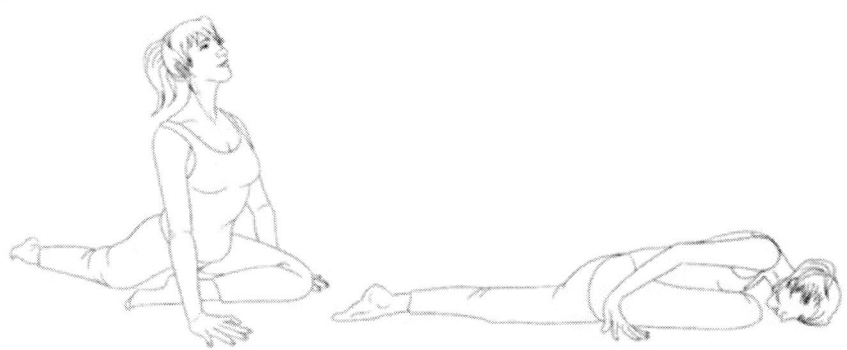

Starting in pigeon pose slowly lower your head and chest to the ground by walking your hands forward.

If you cannot put your head on the ground support it with your hands on between it and the floor.

When ready walk your hands back up until you are back in pigeon pose.

EXTENDED SIDE ANGLE

Avoid if you have a hip, knee, neck, and/or shoulder injury.

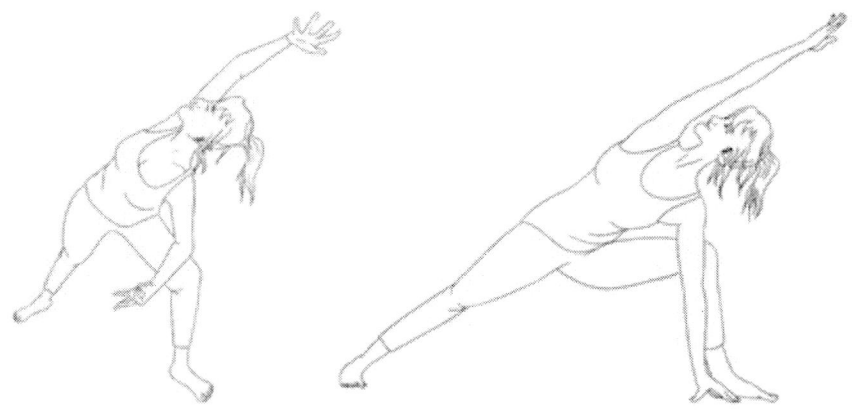

Adopt warrior two, left foot forward, with your left elbow resting on your right knee.

As you inhale raise your right arm to the sky and then as you exhale lengthen it over your ear so that the right side of your body is a straight line.

You could also bring your left hand to the ground on either side of your foot.

Allow your hips to sink to the ground as you reach through your right fingers. Ensure your left knee is directly over your left ankle.

FISH POSE

Avoid if you have an arm, back, neck, and/or shoulder injury.

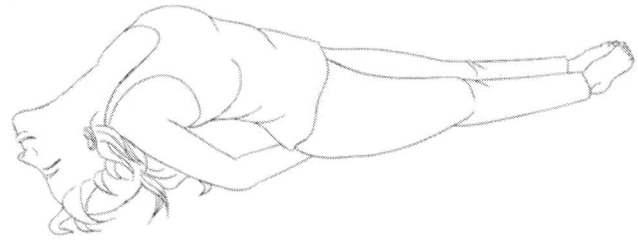

Lie on you back with your legs slightly apart and your arms along the side of your body.

Slide your hands under the top of your thighs. Your elbows are slightly bent out the sides of your torso.

Roll onto the crown of your head by pressing your arms into the ground as you arch your spine and lift your chest.

Place little to no weight on your head and neck. Let the rest of your body do the work.

FIVE POINTED STAR

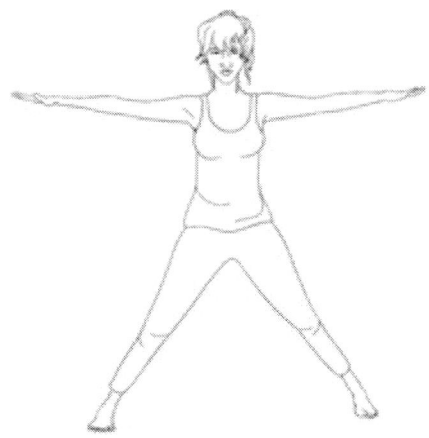

Starting from mountain pose, raise your arms out to the sides and step your feet wide apart so that they are under your wrists and facing forward.

Press your weight down into your feet and strengthen your legs solid into the floor.

Relax your shoulders down and back as you push your chest forward.

As you inhale extend your body up through your crown, down through your feet, and out through your hands.

GATE POSE
Avoid if you have a hip, knee, and/or shoulder injury.

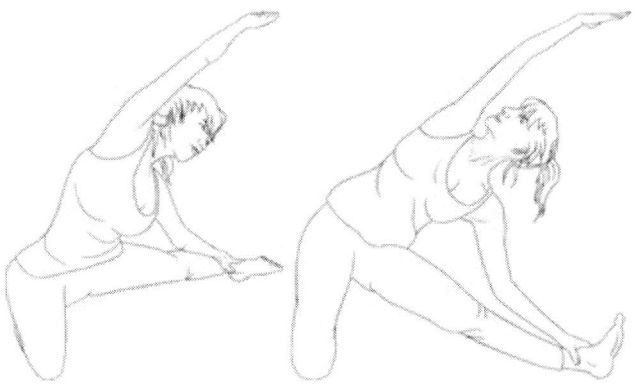

Kneel down with your knees hip width apart.

Straighten your left leg out to your left, foot flat on the ground and toes pointing to the left. Rest your left palm on your left leg.

As you inhale raise your right arm to the sky.

As you exhale drop your right arm over your ear as you slide your left arm to your toes. Keep your arms straight.

Lengthen your body by pressing out through your right hip, pushing into your foot and knee, and reaching out through your fingers and the crown of your head. Keep your chest open and either look straight ahead or up to the sky.

When ready, as you inhale bring your right arm and knee back to a kneeling position.

HALF BOW

Avoid if you have an arm, hip, leg, and/or neck injury, and/or have had recent abdominal surgery, and/or are pregnant.

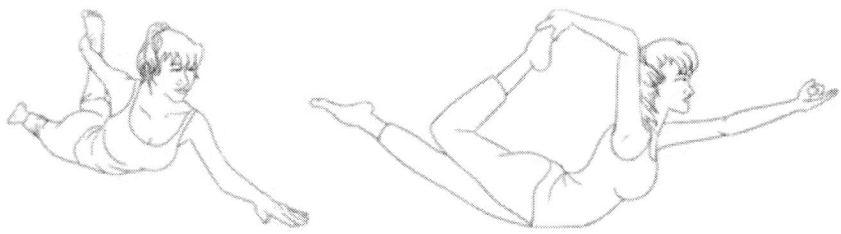

Lie on your stomach with your chin on the floor and your hands over your head, palms facing down. Have your legs either together or just a little apart.

Bend your left knee and grab onto your ankle or heel with your right hand.

As you inhale lift your left leg, chest, and head off the ground. Ensure your neck is in line with your spine and look to your third eye.

Your left arm can either be on the ground in front of you or lifted in the air, parallel to the ground.

When ready exhale as you let your body sink back into the ground.

HALF CAMEL

Avoid if you have a back, knee, neck, and/or shoulder injury, and/or have had recent abdominal surgery, and/or have a hernia.

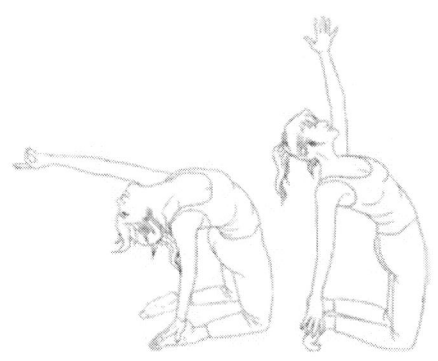

Get on your knees with your palms on your sacrum, fingers pointing to the ground. Ensure your knees are hip width apart. Your feet can either be flat or with your toes tucked.

As you inhale lengthen your spine by pushing the crown of your head to the sky while pressing your knees down.

Press your hips forward and bend backwards as you exhale.

Use your arms to support your weight and very carefully grab your right heel or foot with your right hand. If it is too challenging to grab your foot you can keep your hand on your sacrum.

As you inhale reach your left hand behind you, and if you are comfortable to do so, gently drop your head back. If that is too challenging you can point your hand to the sky.

When ready place both hands back on your sacrum and inhale as you come back to a kneeling position. Bring your head and neck up last.

HALF CIRCLE

Avoid if you have an arm, hip, knee, and/or shoulder injury, and/or you have a hernia.

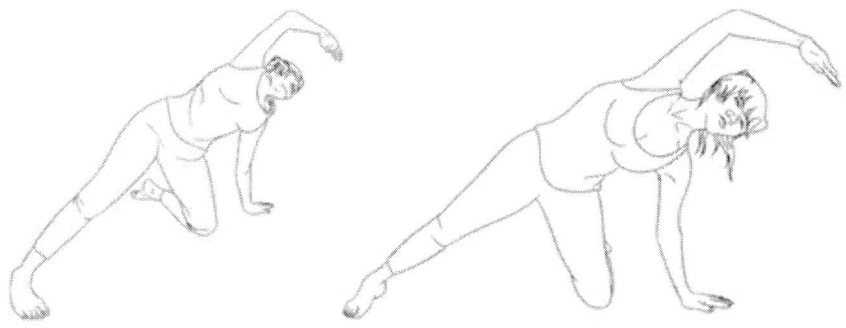

Kneel down with your knees hip width apart.

Straighten your right leg to the side, foot flat on the floor, and toes facing forwards.

Gently lower your left hand to the ground so it is directly under your left shoulder.

As you inhale bring your right hand over your head, palm facing the ground.

Arch your spine as you push your hips forward and let your head drop back.

Reach out through your left fingers as you push your left foot into the ground. The left side of your body makes a half-circle shape.

When you are ready bring your arms parallel to the floor as you inhale, and then as you exhale bring your hands to your hips and step back into a kneeling position.

HALF FORWARD FOLD
Avoid if you have a back, hip, and/or shoulder injury.

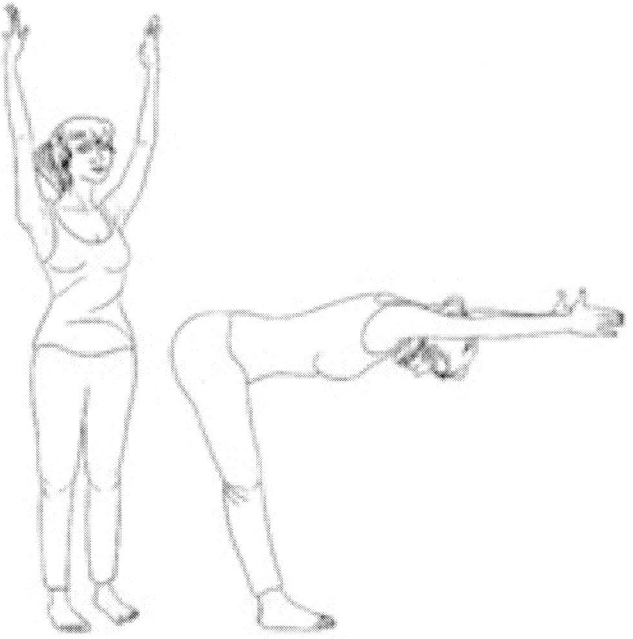

Stand in mountain pose with your palms facing each other.

As you exhale bend forward at your hips until your torso is parallel with the ground. Keep a flat back as you do this.

Lengthen your hips back and your crown and fingers forward. Keep your legs strong.

HALF LOCUST

Avoid if you have a back and/or leg injury, and/or have had recent abdominal surgery, and/or are pregnant.

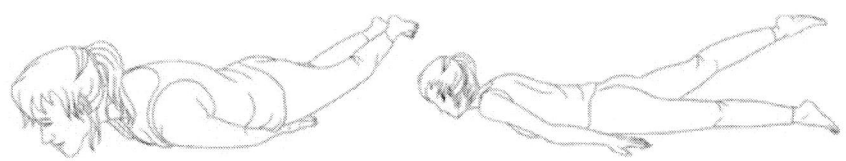

Start by lying on your belly, legs together, and your arms relaxed along the side of your body, palms facing the ground. Rest your chin on the floor.

Bring your hands under your body so that they are under your thighs and with your forearms on the inside of your hips bones. It may help to rock your body from side to side as you inch your arms in. If this is too uncomfortable you can leave your arms alongside your body.

As you inhale lengthen your legs and toes back. Engage your pelvic area and your upper legs as you press your arms into the ground and lift them up to the sky. If that is too challenging just lift one leg at a time.

When ready exhale as you gently relax back to the ground. Turn your head to one side and bring your arms out from under your body.

HALF PRAYER TWIST

Avoid if you have a back, hip, knee, and/or shoulder injury.

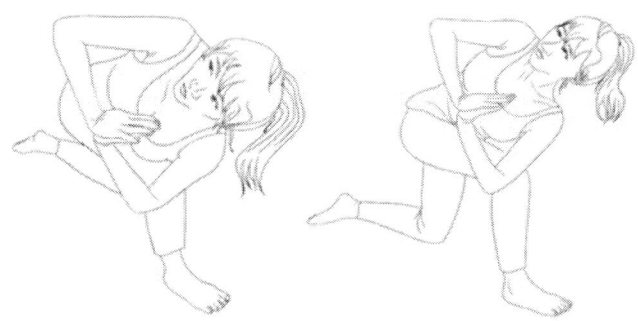

Start in low warrior with your right foot forward and your palms on the floor, one on each side of your front foot.

As you inhale bring your torso up and place your hands together in a prayer position.

Place your right elbow to the outside of your left knee and use your arms to press your right shoulder up and back. Feel it twist your upper back.

Ensure your palms remain in the center of your chest with your fingers pointing towards your throat.

You can either look straight ahead or up towards the sky.

When ready exhale as you bring your palms back to the floor, one on each side of your right foot.

HALF PYRAMID

Avoid if you have a knee, and/or leg injury.

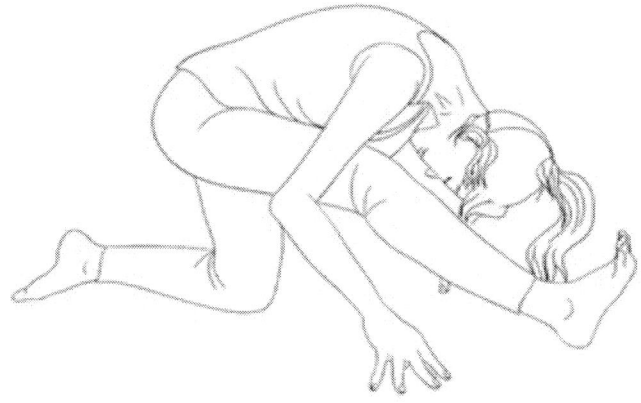

Start in low warrior. While exhaling straighten your right leg as you press your hips back towards your left heel.

Round your spine and lift your toes to the sky as you push your forehead to your right knee. Walk your hands back towards you to support your torso. Relax your elbows, face, neck, and shoulders.

When ready inhale and bend your right knee back over your ankle and then exhale and bring your right knee back into table pose.

HALF SHOULDER-STAND

Avoid if you have a back, neck, and/or shoulder injury, and/or are menstruating or pregnant, and/or have unmediated high blood pressure.

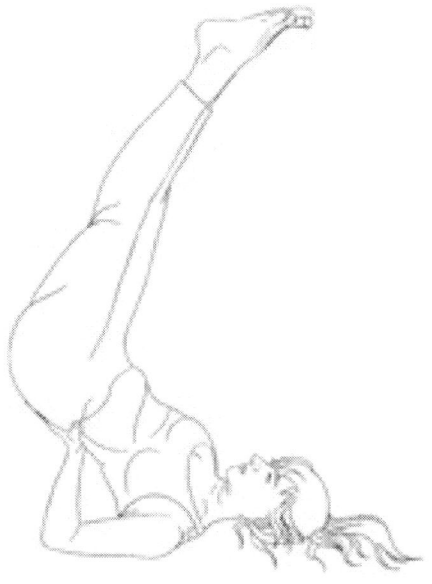

Lie on your back and place your arms along the sides of your body, palms facing down.

Bend your knees and rock back to bring them to your forehead. As you do this place your hands under your hips and cup them for support.

Lift your legs up to straighten them over your head.

You should have very little weight on your head and neck. Support yourself with your arms.

Find the position where you are balanced and then relax your legs.

When ready bend your knees to your head and gently roll your spine back onto the floor.

HALF SUPINE HERO

Avoid if you have a knee injury.

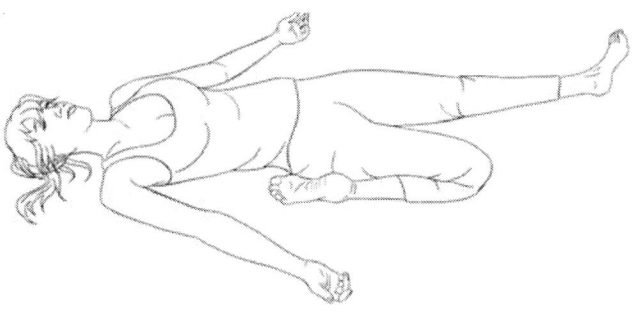

Starting in hero pose extend your left leg in front of you.

Carefully walk your hands behind you and lower your back to the floor. First on your elbows, then the crown of your head, and eventually onto the back of your neck. Only go as low as you feel comfortable.

Once on your back rest your hands down the side of your body.

When you are ready grab you right foot with your right hand and apply pressure to slowly bring yourself back up to a seated position.

HALF UPRIGHT SEATED ANGLE
Avoid if you have a hip, knee, and/or shoulder injury.

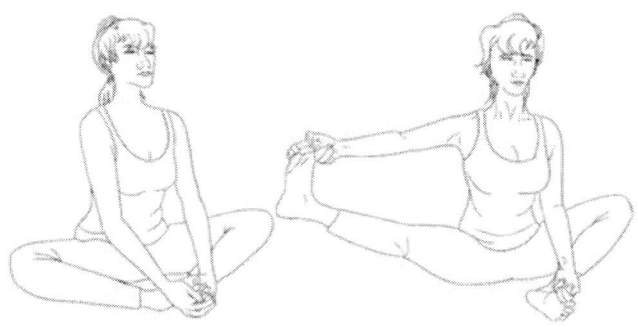

From bound angle pose grab your big toes with the middle and index finger of each hand.

As you inhale lift your right foot off the floor and straighten it to your right. Press out through your heel.

Keep your torso vertical by gently pulling on your left foot.

Push your chest forward and relax your shoulders down and back.

When ready exhale as you bend your right knee and bring your feet back to bound angle pose.

HALF WIND RELIEVING POSE

Avoid if you have a hernia and/or have had recent abdominal surgery.

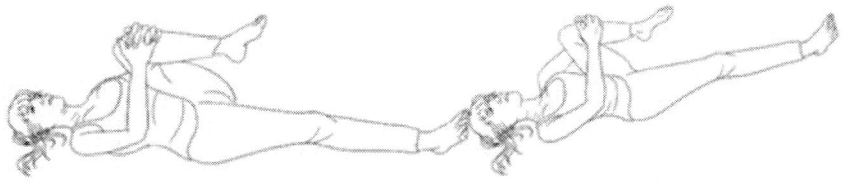

Lie on your back.

As you inhale bring your right knee to your chest and hold it there by interlacing your fingers around it just below the kneecap.

Tuck your chin to your chest with your head on the floor and gently pull your right knee into your chest. Avoid your rib cage when doing this.

Keep your elbows close to your body and push your shoulders and the back of your neck into the floor. Relax your lower body.

As you inhale press your belly into your thigh.

When ready release everything to the floor as you exhale.

HERO POSE
Avoid if you have a knee injury.

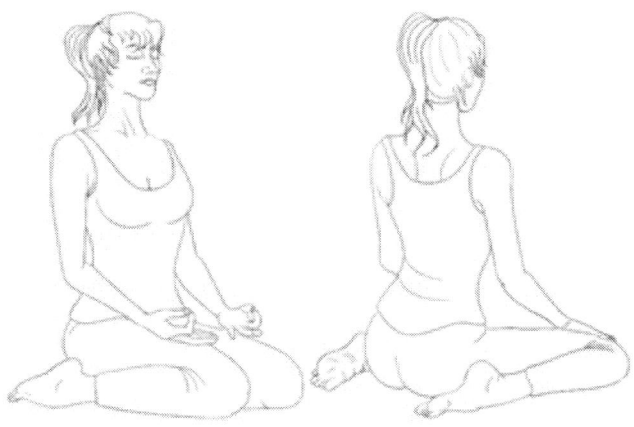

Kneel on the ground with your knees together and your feet hip width apart. Sit with your bum on the ground and your heels on the outside of your hips.

If this is too difficult you can sit on your heels.

Place your hands on your knees. Your palms can face up or down.

Lengthen your torso by reaching the crown of your head to the sky.

Push your lower legs into the ground, drop your shoulders, and press your chest forward.

Relax your belly, face, jaw, and tongue.

Hero pose is an excellent pose to rest and/or for meditation.

HIGH PLANK

Avoid if you have an arm, back, and/or shoulder injury.

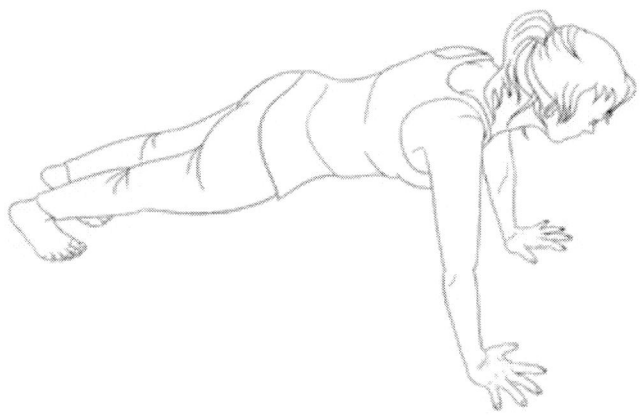

Go into the "up" position of a push up. Spread your fingers wide apart, middle finger facing forward, and press your hands into the ground.

Have straight arms but not locked at the elbow. Tense your bum so that your body forms a straight line.

Push back into your heels as you lengthen through the crown of your head.

JOYFUL BABY
Avoid if you have a leg, neck, and/or shoulder injury.

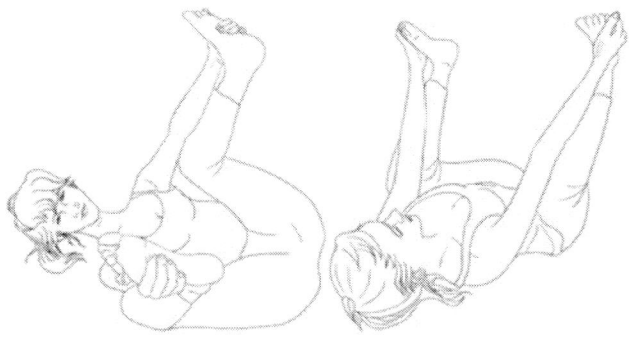

Start in corpse pose.

As you inhale bring your knees to your chest.

Weave your arms through the inside of your knees and hold onto the pinkie toe side edges of your feet with your hands.

Keep your head on the ground and tuck your chin to your chest.

Push your heels up to the sky as you pull back with your arms. At the same time press the back of your neck, shoulders, sacrum, and tailbone to the floor.

Open your legs wider for a deeper hip stretch.

When you are ready exhale and slowly roll your spine back to the ground until you are lying flat again.

KNEE DOWN TWIST
Avoid if you have a back, hip, and/or knee injury.

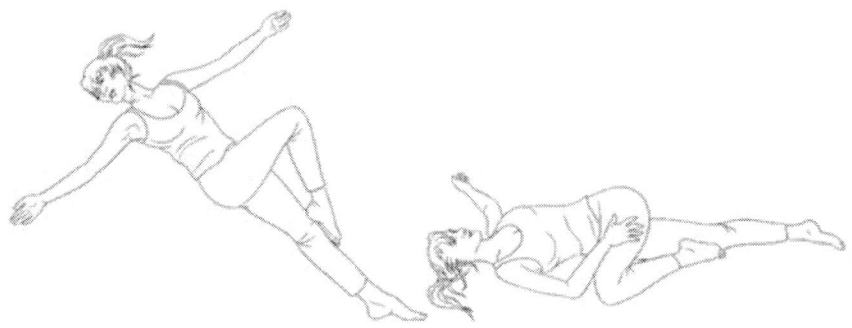

Lie on your back and extend your arms out to your sides at right angles to your torso, palms facing down.

Bend your right knee and place your right foot over your left knee.

As you exhale twist your lower body to the left and allow your right knee to drop over your left leg.

Look to your right fingers or straight up. Relax into the posture allowing gravity to do the work.

For more of a stretch you can put your left hand on your right knee to add more weight. You do not need to push down on it.

When you are ready inhale as you untwist to a straight back and exhale as you lower your leg down to the floor.

LION POSE

Avoid if you have a face, knee, neck, and/or tongue injury.

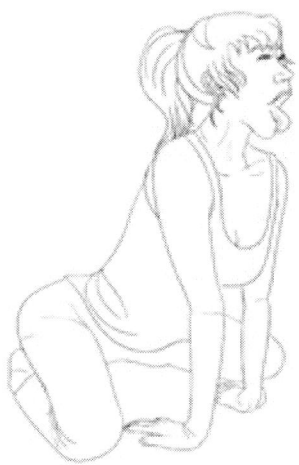

From hero pose bring your feet together and spread your knees as wide as you comfortably can.

Sit on your heels.

Inhale and lengthen your spine by reaching the crown of your head to the sky.

Bring your palms to the floor in between your knees with your fingers facing your body.

Arch your spine, stick your tongue out, and exhale via your mouth ferociously.

Repeat this a few times.

LOW WARRIOR

Avoid if you have an ankle, arm, hip, and/or shoulder injury.

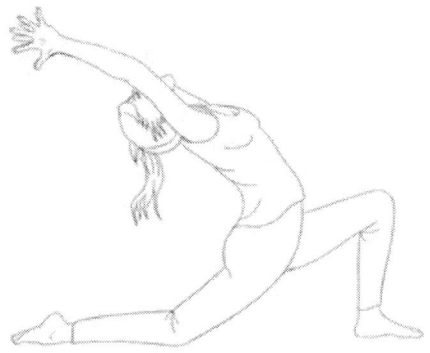

Start in table pose.

Step your right foot forward placing it in-between your hands. Your knee is directly over your ankle.

Ensure your left knee and left and right feet are firm with the ground and then place your hands on your right knee.

Straighten your arms and bring your torso back. Do not lock your elbows.

Relax your shoulders and stick your chest out by bringing your shoulder blades towards each other.

As you inhale raise your arms over your head with your palms facing each other and arch your back as you look up to the sky.

If this is difficult then you can keep your hands on your bent knee.

When ready exhale as you bring your palms back to the floor on either side of your right foot.

MOUNTAIN POSE
Avoid if you have a shoulder injury.

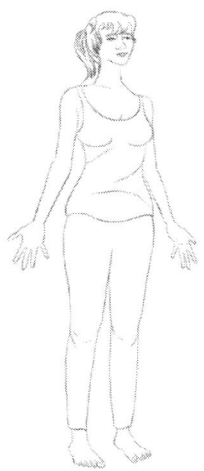

Stand with your feet parallel and either together or hip width apart.

Spread your toes wide and balance your weight evenly and central over each foot.

Pull up your kneecaps and tense your thighs. Keep your legs straight but do not lock your knees.

Ensure your hips are directly over your ankles.

As you inhale lengthen your spine so that the crown of your head goes straight up towards the sky.

When you exhale drop your shoulders and lengthen your finger-tips towards the ground whilst still extending your head upwards.

At the same time gently direct your chest straight ahead.

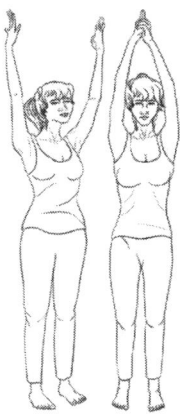

While continuing to lengthen through your finger-tips, inhale and bring your arms up above your head to reach for the sky, palms facing each other.

As you exhale relax your shoulders, but continue to lengthen your crown and fingers to the sky.

An alternative position is to interlace your fingers with your index fingers pointing up.

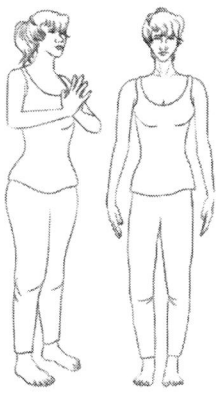

When you are ready exhale and bring your palms together in front of your chest in a prayer position. Take a breath and on the exhale allow your hands to drop to your sides.

ONE HANDED TIGER

Avoid if you have a back, hip, knee, and/or shoulder injury.

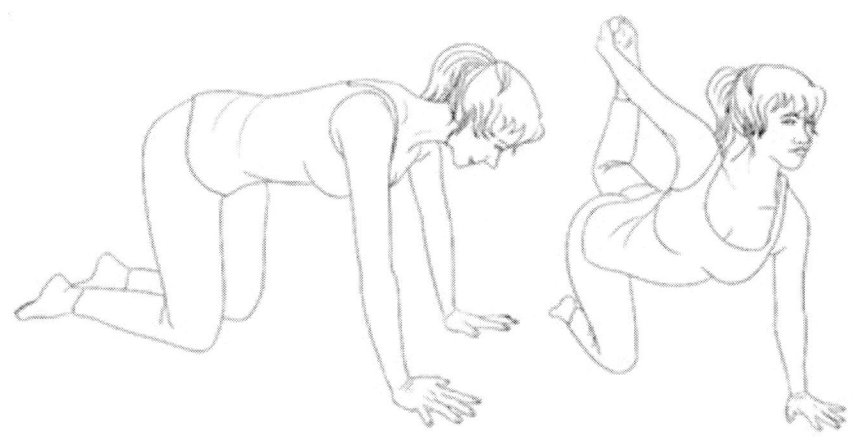

Start in table pose.

As you exhale, keeping your knee bent and gently arching your spine, extend your left foot to the sky.

Put your weight over your left hand and use your right hand to hold onto the inside of your left foot or ankle.

Keep both arms straight and look straight ahead. Gently lift your left leg higher.

When ready exhale as you return to table pose.

ONE LEGGED DOLPHIN

Avoid if you have an arm, back, and/or shoulder injury, and/or have glaucoma, and/or unmediated high blood pressure.

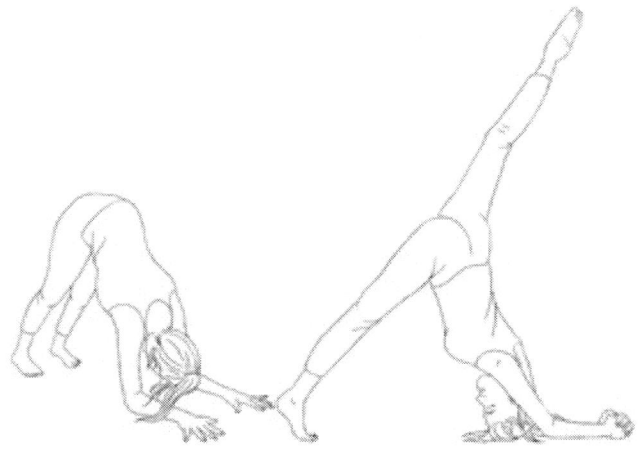

Starting from dolphin pose interlace your fingers together and raise one leg to the sky.

Stretch out through both your feet, i.e., one into the ground and the other towards sky.

PIGEON POSE

Avoid if you have a back, hip, and/or knee injury.

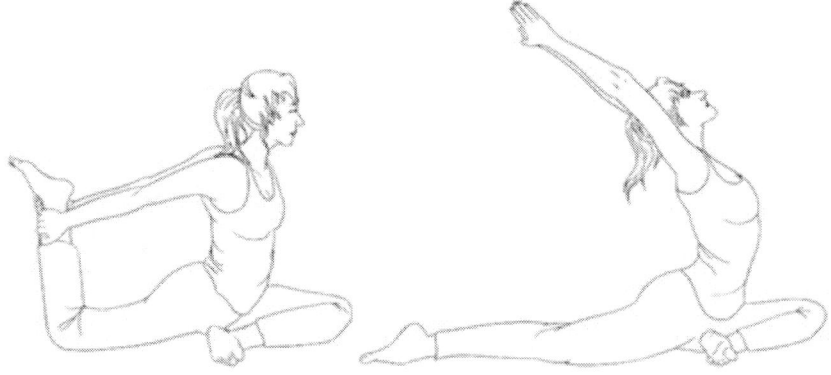

From table or downward dog slide your left knee between your hands and allow your left foot to slide to over to the right.

Shift your right leg back and lower your hips towards the ground.

As you inhale press into your hands and lengthen your spine by pressing the crown of your head to the sky. Drop your hips into the ground as you exhale. Push out through your chest and roll your shoulders back and down.

To increase the stretch slide your left foot further away from your hips.

A couple of variations include lifting up your right lower leg and reaching back with your arms to grab your right ankle, or to bring your hands above your head in a prayer position (or some other mudra) whilst arching your back.

PRAYER SQUAT
Avoid if you have a hip and/or knee injury.

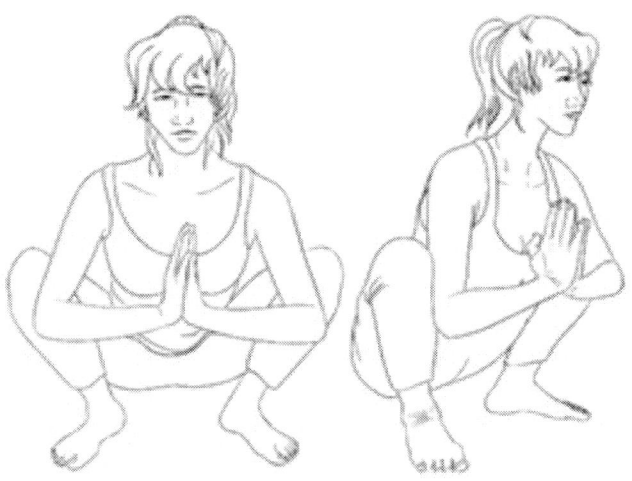

From mountain pose put your palms together in front of your chest in a prayer position. Spread your legs about hip width apart and squat all the way down.

Shift your feet a little further apart if needed until your torso is not resting on your thighs. If you are able have your feet flat on the ground.

Lengthen your spine by sinking your hips to the ground as your reach the crown of your head to the sky. Push your chest forwards and roll your shoulders down and back.

If you can do so without losing balance close your eyes and look to your third eye.

PYRAMID POSE

Avoid if you have a back, hip, and/or shoulder injury.

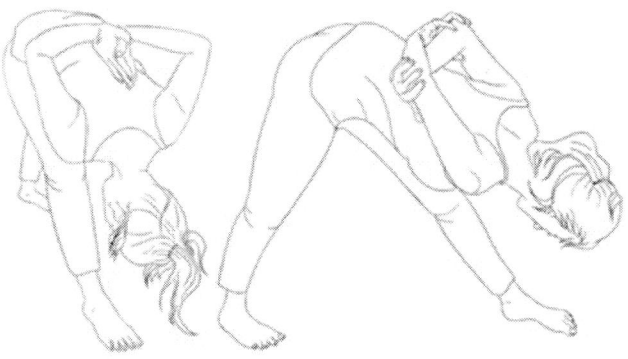

Start with your left foot forward in warrior one.

Step back with your right foot to straighten both of your legs. Make sure your rear foot is flat with your toes facing forwards.

Push your forehead towards your left knee as you press the back of your knees and your heels to your rear.

If you are able bring your hands behind your back either in a prayer position or holding onto your elbows.

RABBIT POSE

Avoid if you have a knee, neck, shoulder, and/or spine injury.

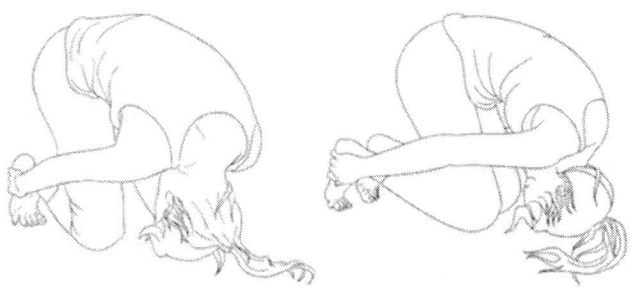

From child pose grab onto your heels and place the top of your head on the ground. Pull your forehead to your knees.

As you inhale lift your hips to the sky.

Roll onto the crown of your head and try to get your forehead as close to your knees as you can.

SEATED ANGLE

Avoid if you have an arm, hip, knee, and/or shoulder injury.

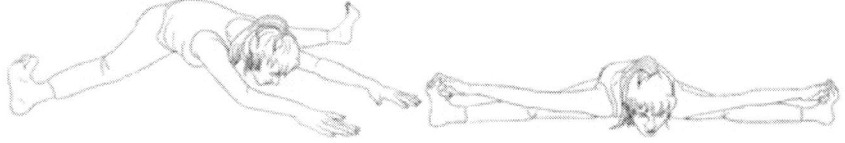

Start in staff pose.

As you inhale spread your legs out as wide as comfortable.

Ensure your knees and toes are pointing up and reach through your fingers up to the sky.

Exhale as you lower your palms to the floor.

Deepen the stretch by walking your hands forward. Stay focused on keeping your spine long.

You could also hold your big toes and use them to help pull your torso down.

When ready inhale and slowly walk your hands in as your roll back your spine until finishing with a straight back.

SEATED FORWARD BEND

Avoid if you have an ankle, arm, hip, and/or shoulder injury.

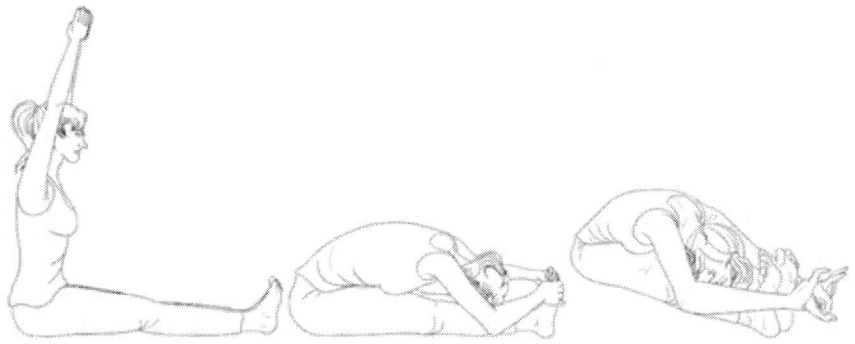

Begin in staff pose.

Inhale and raise your arms up to the sky with your palms facing each other. Lengthen your torso through your fingers and the crown of your head.

As you exhale bend at the hips, lowering your upper body to your legs. Grab your ankles, feet, or toes.

Push out through your heels as you pull your toes back towards you.

You can use your arms to pull yourself closer to your legs. For those with more flexibility reach your hands in front of your feet.

If you are having difficulties bend your knees enough so you can reach your feet and place your head on your knees.

When you are ready slowly roll up your spine back into staff pose.

SEATED HEAD TO KNEE
Avoid if you have a back and/or knee injury.

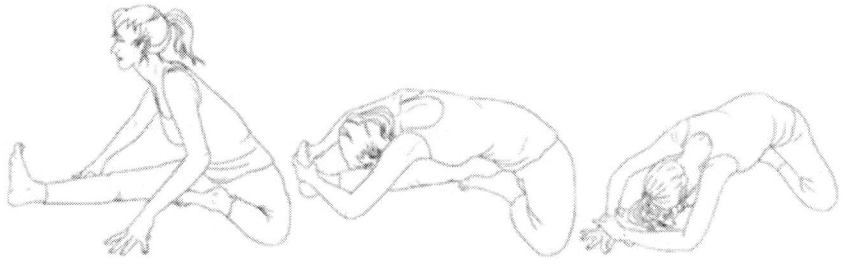

Start in bound angle and extend your right leg out in front of you. Put the bottom of your left foot up against your right thigh and have your hips square.

As you inhale raise your arms up and lengthen your spine through the crown of your head and your fingertips.

Continue to lengthen as you exhale and bend forward at your hips. Interlace your fingers around your right foot. Bend your knee if you need to.

Press your head down into your knee and push your right heel away from you in an effort to straighten your leg. Pull your toes back towards you.

Relax your upper body. Only use your arms as much as needed to keep your head in contact with your knee.

To increase the stretch reach your hands past your foot and grab your wrist.

When ready inhale your arms back over your head and then exhale as you bring them to the ground.

SEATED SPINAL TWIST
Avoid if you have a back, hip, and/or shoulder injury.

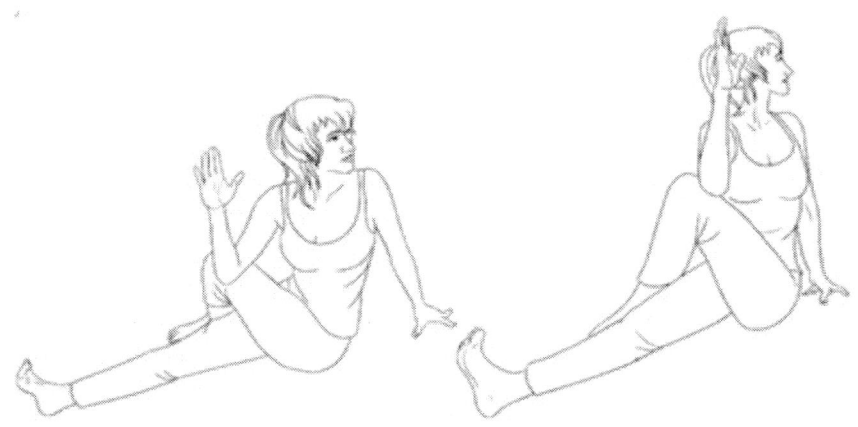

From staff pose cross your left leg over your right and place your left foot flat on the floor near your right knee.

Wrap your right arm around your left knee and pull it into your chest. Lengthen your spine by pushing up through the crown of your head and down through your waist.

As you inhale raise your left hand up and then exhale as you place it on the ground behind you, fingers facing back. Keep your back straight by pressing your arm into it.

Look over your left shoulder as you place your right elbow on the outside of your left knee.

Inhale and lengthen your spine. As you exhale use your arms to increase the twist. Relax your shoulders and push your chest out to open it.

When ready inhale as you lift your left hand up and untwist your body to face forwards.

SIDE SEATED ANGLE

Avoid if you have a hip, leg, and/or lower back injury.

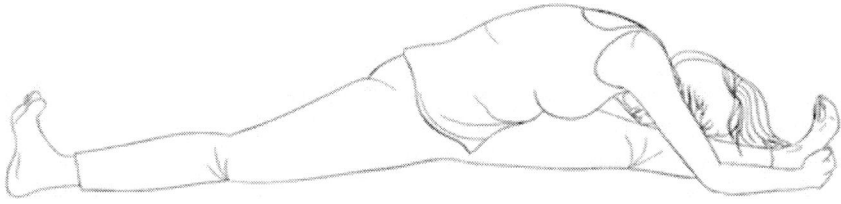

Start in seated angle.

Turn to face your right foot by twisting at your waist.

Walk your hands towards your right foot as you exhale. Try to reach your forehead to your knee and hold your right ankle or foot if you are able.

Relax your shoulders and neck and then increase the stretch by pressing your heel out while pulling your toes back towards yourself.

When ready return to the center with your back straight and then do the same thing on your left side.

STAFF POSE

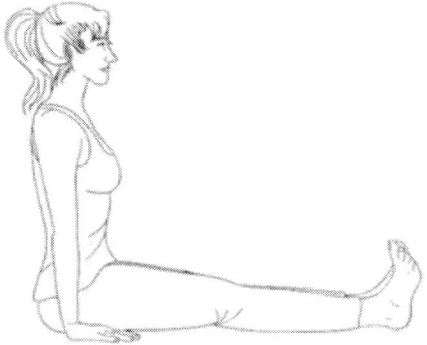

Move into a seated position with your legs extended straight out in front of you. Place your hands beside your hips with your fingers pointed forward.

Lengthen your spine by pressing your hip bones down whilst pushing the crown of your head towards the sky. Use your arms for support as you push your chest forward and lower your shoulders.

Pull your toes towards your head as you push your heels away from you.

STANDING BACK BEND

Avoid if you have a back, hip, and/or neck injury.

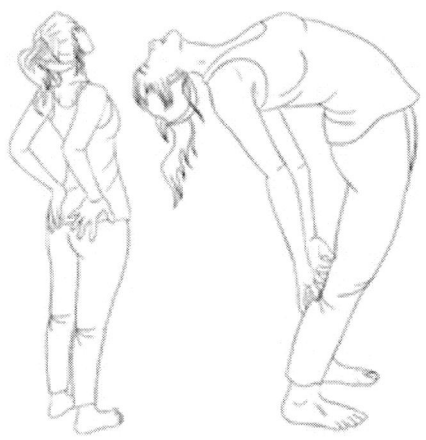

Begin in mountain pose.

As you breathe in place the palms of your hands on your lower back (sacrum) with your fingers pointing to the ground.

Squeeze your buttocks and thighs tight, pull up your knee caps, and press into your feet.

Exhale and press your hips forward as you arch your back.

You can either look straight ahead or allow your head to drop all the way back.

Increase the stretch by walking your hands down the back of your legs.

When you are ready slowly come back to a standing position with your hands by your sides.

STANDING FORWARD FOLD

Avoid if you have a back, hip, leg, and/or shoulder injury.

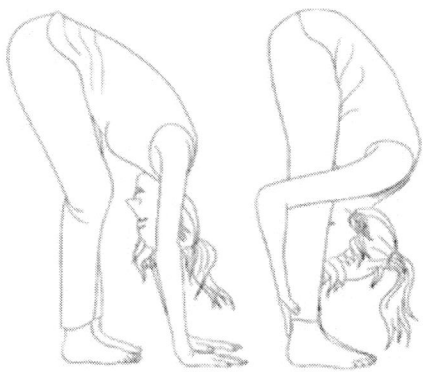

Being in mountain position.

Exhale and bring your head to your knees with your palms flat on the floor.

Stretch your spine by pulling your head down while pushing your hips up.

Bend your knees if you need to but continuously aim to be able to do it with straight legs.

Press your belly into your thighs when inhaling.

For a deeper stretch hold the back of your calves and pull your head closer to your legs.

STANDING YOGA SEAL

Avoid if you have a back, leg, neck, and/or shoulder injury, and/or unmediated high blood pressure.

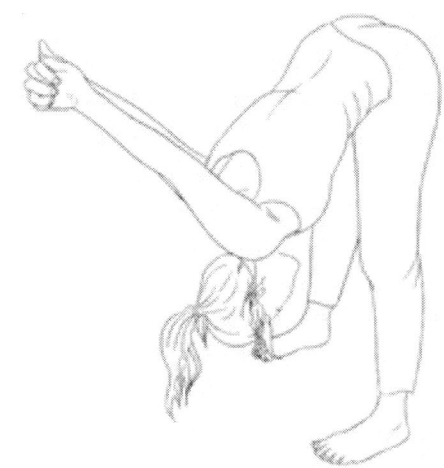

From five pointed star inhale as you interlace your fingers behind you.

Draw your shoulders back to expand your chest and look up to the sky.

As you exhale keep your legs and arms straight and bend forward at your hips.

Reach your arms up and forward and allow your head to hang.

Keep your weight even over your feet.

To make the pose harder bring your feet closer together.

When ready inhale as you come back up and exhale as you release your arms.

SUPINE BOUND ANGLE

Avoid if you have a hip and/or shoulder injury.

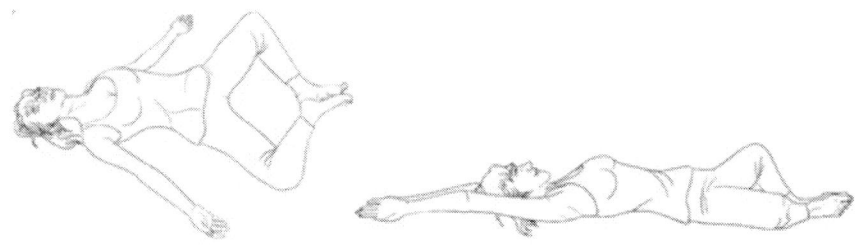

From corpse pose bend your legs to bring the bottoms of your feet together.

Your knees bend facing out just like in bound angle but lying down. Allow your knees to drop to the ground.

You can rest your hands on your thighs to "encourage" them but do not push down.

As you inhale slide your arms on the ground over your head until your palms are together. Cross your thumbs.

When ready exhale as you return to a lying position.

TABLE POSE

Avoid if you have a knee and/or wrist injury.

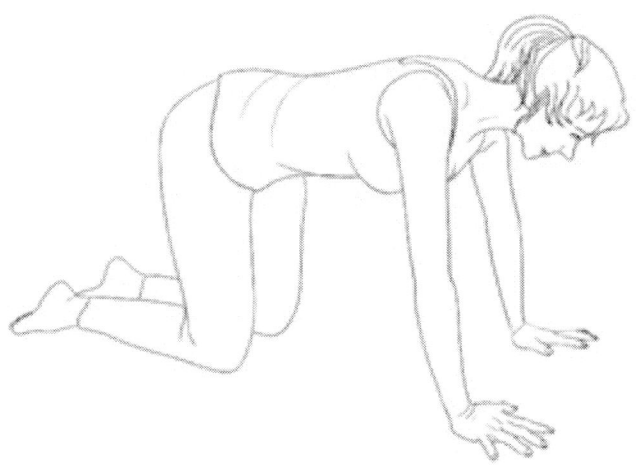

As you inhale place your hands and knees on the floor with your palms directly underneath your shoulders and fingers facing forwards.

Ensure your knees are shoulder width apart and your feet are directly behind them with the tops of your feet and toes on the floor.

Look at the ground between your hands and press down into your palms.

Have your back flat and exhale while lengthening your spine by pressing the crown of your head forward and your tailbone back.

THREADING THE NEEDLE

Avoid if you have a knee, neck, and/or shoulder injury.

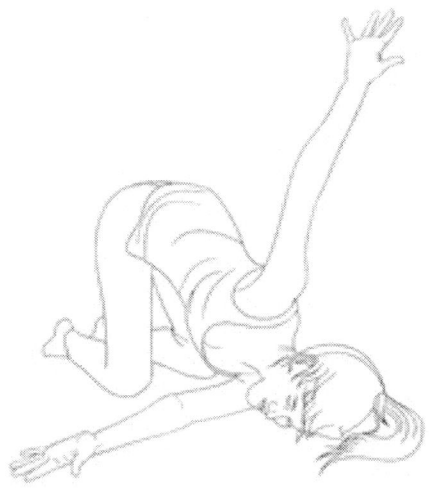

Start in table pose.

As you exhale slide your right hand between your left knee and left hand until your right shoulder and the side of your head are resting on the floor.

Inhale and reach towards the sky with your left hand.

Find where you get the deepest stretch and stay there, reaching out through your fingers.

When ready exhale as you bring your hand back to the floor and then inhale to readopt table pose.

Repeat on your left side.

TREE POSE
Avoid if you have a hip and/or knee injury.

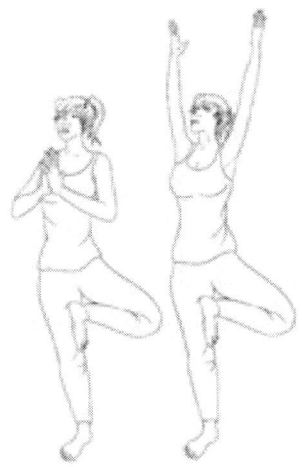

Stand in mountain pose and then shift all your weight over your right leg.

Bend your left knee so that your left heel rests on your right leg.

Slide your left foot up your right leg as high as you can without losing balance. Point your toes to the ground.

Bring your hands together in prayer position.

Press your chest forward and your right foot into the ground.

If you are able inhale and bring your hands above your head, palms facing each other. Reach up through your fingers.

When ready exhale as your return to mountain pose.

TRIANGLE POSE
Avoid if you have a back, hip, and/or shoulder injury.

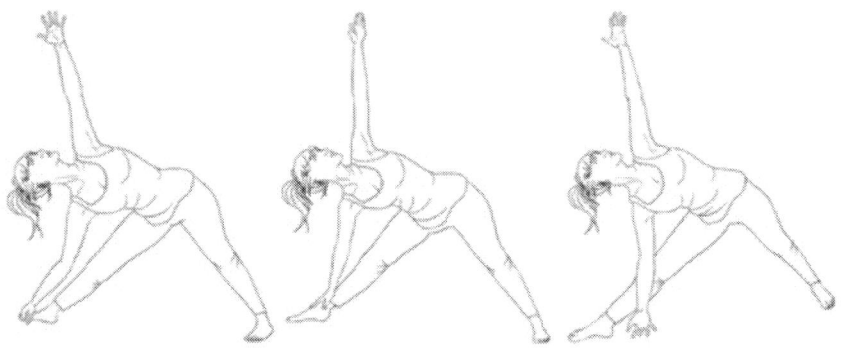

From five pointed star point your right toes to your right and turn your left toes slightly inwards.

As you inhale push your hip to the left and slide your arms to the right so they are parallel to the floor.

Rotate your arms as you exhale, resting your right hand against your right leg and raising your left arm up, palms facing forward.

Make a straight line with your arms and stretch out through your fingertips. Press your feet into the ground.

Your right hand can either be on your ankle, grabbing your toes, or on the ground.

When you are ready inhale as you return to five pointed star.

UPWARD BOAT

Avoid if you have an abdomen, hip, knee, and/or shoulder injury.

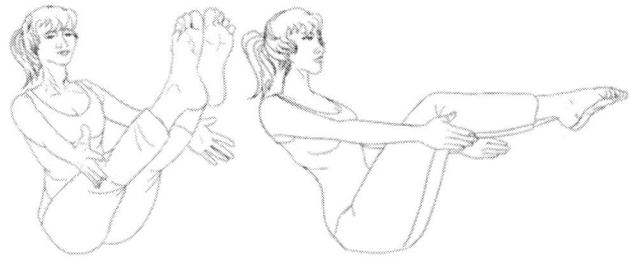

Sit down on your bum with your knees bent and feet flat on the floor.

Put your legs together and place your hands behind your hips with your elbows bent away from you and your fingers pointing forwards.

Lift your heels off the ground a little by leaning back.

Open your chest by drawing your shoulder blades together.

Slowly straighten your legs and lift them as high as you are comfortable.

Extend your arms forwards palms facing the floor and parallel to the ground.

Continue to lift your chest with the same amount of effort as you use to lift your legs.

If this is to challenging keep your knees bent and/or your hands on the floor.

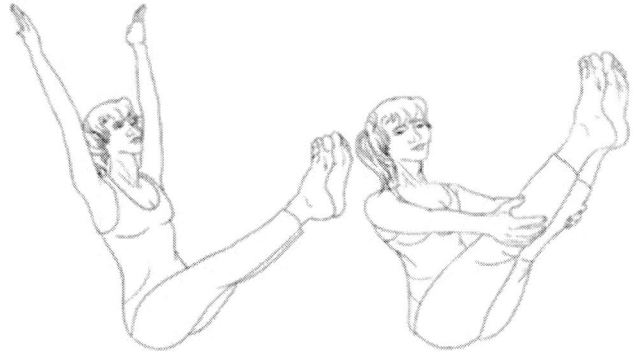

You can also reach both your hands above your head or hold onto the back of your knees.

When you are ready exhale as you bend your knees and then lower your feet back to the ground.

UPWARD DOG

Avoid if you have an arm, back, hip, and/or shoulder injury, and/or have had recent abdominal surgery, and/or are pregnant.

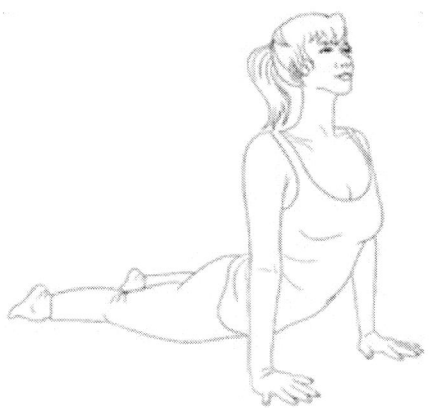

From table pose drop your hips forward towards the ground as you press your palms down into the floor.

Press your chest forward as you drop your shoulders down and back.

Push the crown of your head towards the ceiling.

As you inhale press the tops of your feet into the ground to lift your legs off the floor.

Only the tops of your feet and your hands touch the ground.

Press all of your toenails firmly into the floor.

UPWARD FORWARD FOLD
Avoid if you have an arm, back, and/or shoulder injury.

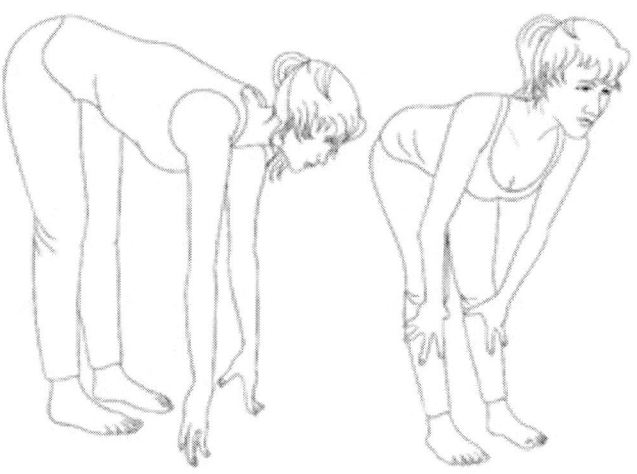

Allow your hands to dangle down to the ground.

Place your hands on the floor if they reach.

As you inhale arch your back and look to the sky.

Extend your nose forward, push your sternum to the floor, and lengthen your tailbone behind you.

If you are having difficulties bring your hands to your knees.

WARRIOR ONE

Avoid if you have a back, hip, knee, and/or shoulder injury.

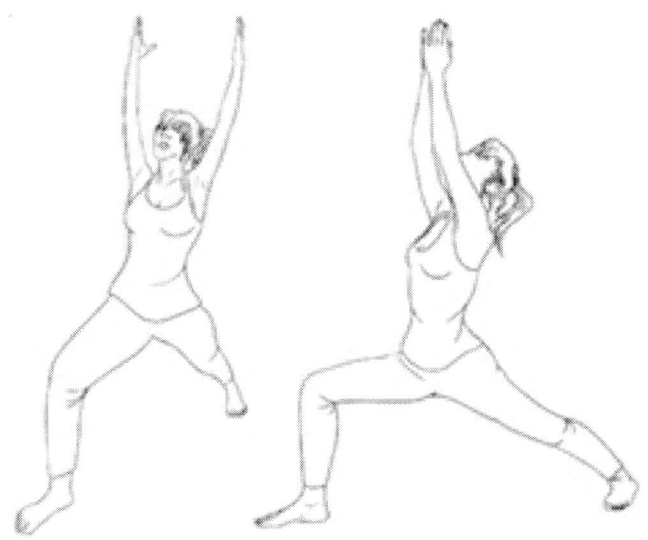

From five pointed star bend your right knee and turn to face your right.

Turn your left foot 45° and keep your heel on the floor. Your front foot heel and the arch of your rear foot are lined up.

Ensure your right knee is directly over your ankle with your hips and shoulders square and facing forwards.

As you inhale raise your arms above your head with your palms facing each other. Keep your shoulders relaxed and your chest lifted.

Go deeper by bringing your palms together and carefully arching your back as you look to the sky.

Press into your feet and extend through your fingers and crown as you exhale.

When ready exhale as you lower your hands down to the floor.

WARRIOR TWO

Avoid if you have a hip, knee, and/or shoulder injury.

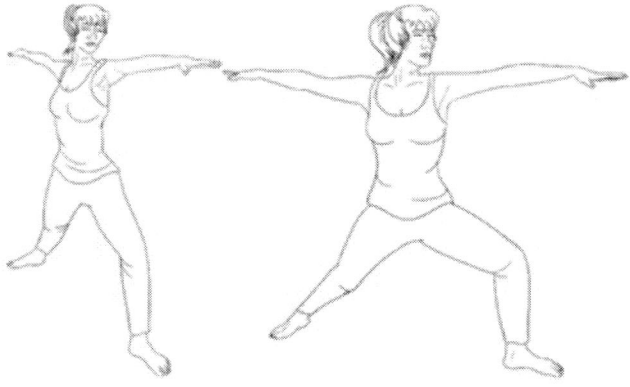

From five pointed star bend your left knee directly over your left ankle, turning your left foot so your toes face to your left.

Keep your right foot planted into the ground as you turn to look to your left fingers.

Push your chest forwards and relax your shoulders.

Lengthen your spine by reaching the crown of your head to the sky and sinking your hips to the ground.

WIDE LEGGED FORWARD BEND

Avoid if you have a back, hip, leg, and/or shoulder injury.

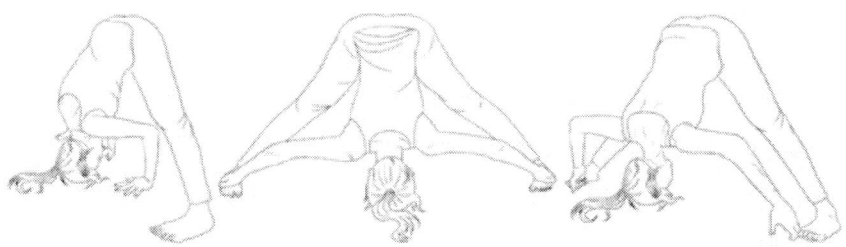

From five pointed star exhale and bend at your waist to bring your palms to the ground under your shoulders.

Keep your back straight.

Widen your legs if you need to in order to make your hands reach the floor.

Bend your elbows to your rear as you pull your forehead towards the ground.

Push your feet into the ground and raise your hips to the sky.

You can also hold onto your feet or toes.

When ready, inhale back up into five pointed star.

WIND RELIEVING POSE

Avoid if you have a hernia and/or have had recent abdominal surgery.

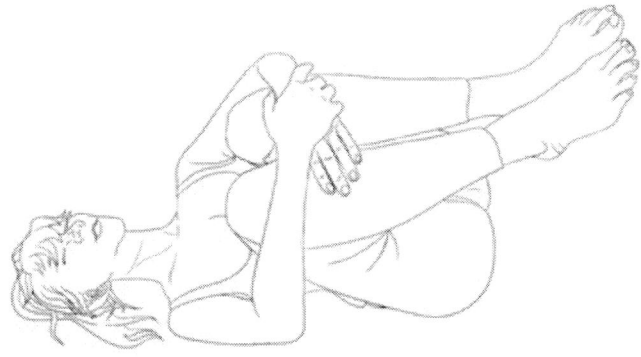

Start in corpse pose.

As you inhale bring both knees up to your chest.

Hug your knees and hold onto your opposite elbows, forearms, fingers, or wrists.

Keep your head on the floor whilst tucking your chin to your chest.

Pull your knees to your chest as you press the back of your neck, shoulders, sacrum, and tailbone to the floor.

Relax your feet, hips, and legs.

Inhale deeply into your belly and press it against your thighs as you do so.

When ready exhale and relax all your limbs to the ground so you are lying flat again.

Dear Reader,

Thank you for reading **Curing Yoga.**

If you enjoyed it, please leave a review on Amazon. It helps more than most people think. You can do that here:

www.SurvivalFitnessPlan.com/Curing-Yoga-Review-Amazon

For any feedback on how to improve this or any of my books you can contact me here:

www.SurvivalFitnessPlan.com/Contact

You can claim your bonus freebies at:

www.SurvivalFitnessPlan.com/Book-Bonus-Freebies

The password is: CYPFS&*98

And you can get FREE training schedules and more by joining our newsletter:

www.SurvivalFitnessPlan.com/Free-Downloads

Thanks again for your support,

Aventuras De Viaje.

AUTHOR RECOMMENDATIONS

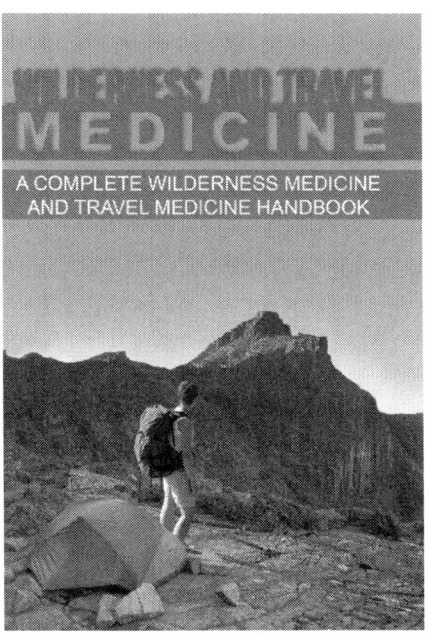

This is the Only Wilderness Medicine Book You Need

Discover what you need to heal yourself, because a little knowledge goes a long way!

Get it now.

www.SurvivalFitnessPlan.com/Wilderness-Travel-Medicine

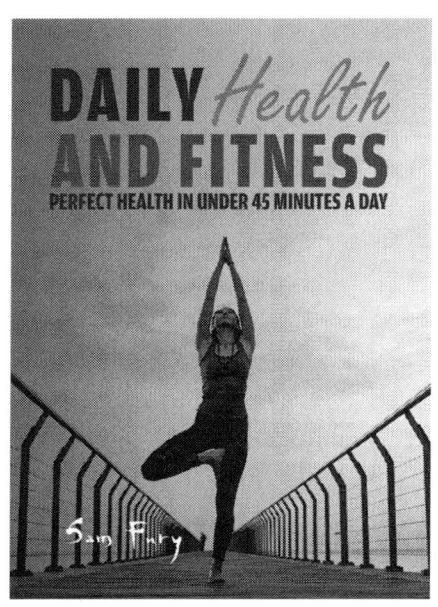

Improve and Maintain Your Health

You'll love this approach to fitness, because it is simple and effective.

Get it now.

www.SurvivalFitnessPlan.com/Daily-Health

SURVIVAL FITNESS PLAN TRAINING MANUALS

Health and Fitness

Keep your body in optimal condition with minimal effort. The health and fitness series covers:

- **Nutrition and conditioning.** The 2 fundamentals for health and fitness.
- **Yoga.** Making Yoga a part of you daily routine will keep your mind and body healthy and in sync. Certain Yoga sequences are also a good alternative cure for many ailments.
- **Massage Therapy.** For prevention and healing of training injuries as well as general relaxation.

www.SurvivalFitnessPlan.com/Health-Fitness-Series

Survival Fitness

When in danger you have two options. Fight or Flight.

This series contains training manuals on the best methods of flight. Together with self defense, you can train in them for general health and fitness.

- **Parkour.** All the parkour skills needed to overcome obstacles in your path.
- **Climbing.** Focusing on essential bouldering techniques.
- **Riding.** Essential mountain bike riding techniques. Go as fast as possible in the safest manner.
- **Swimming.** Swimming for endurance and/or speed using the most efficient strokes.

www.SurvivalFitnessPlan.com/Survival-Fitness-Series

Self Defense

The Self Defense Series has volumes on some of the martial arts used as a base in SFP Self Defense.

It also contains the SFP Self Defense training manuals. SFP Self Defense is an efficient and effective form of minimalist self defense.

www.SurvivalFitnessPlan.com/Self-Defense-Series

Escape Evasion, and Survival

SFP escape, evasion, and survival skills (EES) focus on minimalism. It is EES using little to no special equipment.

- **Escape and Evasion.** The ability to escape capture and hide from your enemy.
- **Urban and Wilderness Survival.** Being able to live off the land in all terrains.
- **Emergency Roping.** Basic climbing skills and improvised roping techniques.
- **Water Rescue.** Life-saving water skills based on surf life-saving and military training course competencies.
- **Wilderness First Aid.** Modern medicine for use in emergency situations.

Specific subjects covered include entry and exit techniques, evasive driving, hostile negotiation tactics, lock-picking, urban survival, wilderness survival, computer hacking, and more.

www.SurvivalFitnessPlan.com/Escape-Evasion-Survival-Series

ABOUT THE AUTHOR

Aventuras has 3 passions: travel, writing, and self-improvement.

Combining these 3 things Miss Viaje spends her time exploring the world and learning about all the things she loves.

She takes what she learns and shares it through her books.

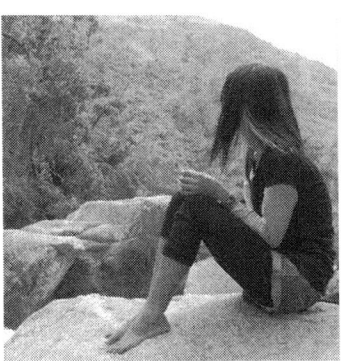

www.SurvivalFitnessPlan.com

facebook.com/SurvivalFitnessPlan

twitter.com/Survival_Fitnes

pinterest.com/survivalfitnes

goodreads.com/MissAventurasDeViaje

amazon.com/author/aventuras

Printed in Great Britain
by Amazon